UNSTOPPABLE

"I remember the morning it came to me that it was time for the people of California to vote on labeling GMOs. The idea came to me unbidden. It washed over me in a full body knowing that did not come from a logical place. It literally made me sit up from my half dream state. I simply knew this was what I was going to do for the next two years. I felt at peace, calm, with the surety of knowing this was The Path.

I was also terrified beyond measure at the enormity of the task.

This all came simultaneously—the peace/calm and the terror. I simply felt both fully in my body. And then I noticed the depression I had been in lifted. I no longer felt paralyzed with fear.

I made two commitments to myself: to be fully willing to look like a fool if this crazy idea went nowhere . . . and that I would not stop unless stopped. There were many points over the following months where it looked like I would, indeed, be stopped. I had to give up all control to something greater than me. And . . . both I and this project just kept going. It's been one of the most amazing rides of my life."

—Pamm Larry, instigator of GMO labeling initiative in California and founder of The Good Food Brigade

"It is my UNSTOPPABLE love for my son, and for all children of the Earth, that has kept me going for the last four decades of ecological activism, beginning with the Chipko movement when peasant women of my region in the Himalaya said they would hug the trees to prevent their logging. Chipko means to embrace, and what could be a more powerful expression of love than the embrace and the hug.

For the last three decades through Navdanya I have embraced the smallest of seeds, the richness of biodiversity, the tiniest of organisms in the soil, the insects and pollinators that control pests and pollinate our crops. My embrace is the practice and promotion of ecological agriculture, an agriculture without poisons, pesticides, or GMOs.

We face a vicious assault on life and freedom from corporations whose only expertise is to kill. They began as companies producing chemical weapons. They retooled the instruments of war as agrochemical inputs, with GMO seeds being the latest in this treadmill of poison."

—Dr. Vandana Shiva, ecofeminist and mother, scientist, ecologist, ecofeminist, founder of the Indian-based nonprofit Navdanya, the movement for seed saving and agroecology

"I am UNSTOPPABLE because our food is our future. Without clean food, healthy food, right out of the ground food that has not been genetically modified, we have no future."

—Joanie, UNSTOPPABLE Mom

UNSTOPPABLE

*To Sarah,
For your Unstoppable
support of health
+ freedom!
♡ Ben Honeycutt*

UNSTOPPABLE

Transforming Sickness and Struggle
into Triumph, Empowerment,
and a Celebration of Community

Zen Honeycutt
Founding Executive Director, Moms Across America

Foreword by
Jill C. Carnahan, MD, ABFM, ABHM, IFMCP
Functional Medicine Practitioner, Conventional Farmer's Daughter,
Breast Cancer and Crohn's Disease Survivor

MOMS ACROSS AMERICA PUBLISHING
Mission Viejo
2018

Copyright © 2018 by Zen LaBossiere Honeycutt.

All rights reserved. No part of this book may be reproduced in any form without the written permission of the publisher.

Published in the United States by Moms Across America Publishing.
Library of Congress Cataloging-in-Publication Data
Honeycutt, Zen LaBossiere.
UNSTOPPABLE: transforming sickness and struggle into triumph, empowerment, and a celebration of community/Zen Honeycutt—1 st ed.
2018903959

ISBN 978-1986668262

Printed in the United States of America
First Printing April 2018

Development and Copy Editor: Debbie Luican
Interior Book Designer: Claudine Mansour Design
Cover Designer: Anne Temple
Photographers: Todd Honeycutt and Marcus Caspian

About Moms Across America Publishing
Moms Across America Publishing is committed to amplifying the voices of truth-telling citizens, especially moms. From our house to yours . . . we champion authors who are honest, kind, and whose information will make a difference for your family. Moms Across America Publishing is a branch of the Moms Across America 501(c)3 nonprofit. A large portion of the proceeds from the sales of our books supports the empowerment and health of families both nationwide and worldwide.

Moms Across America Publishing
24000 Alicia Parkway #17-236
Mission Viejo, CA 92691
info@momsacrossamerica.org

Disclaimer
The contents of this book are presented as helpful information. This book is not meant to be used, nor should it be used, to diagnose or treat any medical condition. For diagnosis or treatment, please consult a medical professional (we suggest integrative medicine). The publisher and author are not responsible for medical conditions requiring professional supervision, nor are they liable for any damage or negative consequences for any specific health actions resulting from reading this book. References are provided for informational purposes only and do not constitute an endorsement of any website or other resource on the part of the authors or publisher. The author or publisher have not been compensated to list any such resources. Readers should be aware that the websites listed in the book might change.

This book is dedicated to:

My mother, Mavis Jan Lai,
who gave me not only life but also the desire to marvel at nature.

My father, Paul William LaBossiere,
who was the first environmentalist in my life and
who taught me I could do anything.

My husband, Todd, and children, Ben, Bodee, and Bronson,
who make this life a wonderful adventure.

CONTENTS

Foreword — xiii
Acknowledgments — xvii
Introduction: Things Have Changed — xix

Part One: UNSTOPPABLE Love
Chapter One: Love in Action — 3
Chapter Two: Learning the Truth about GMOs — 19
Chapter Three: Learning the Truth about Glyphosate — 31

Part Two: UNSTOPPABLE Community
Chapter Four: Trust, Truth, and Community — 61
Chapter Five: A Healthy Community Starts with a Healthy Family — 83
Chapter Six: Toxins in Daily Life — 105

Part Three: UNSTOPPABLE Leadership
Chapter Seven: Activism — 125
Chapter Eight: Stepping into Leadership — 147
Chapter Nine: Speaking to Friends, Family, and Strangers — 165
Chapter Ten: In the Lion's Den — 179
Chapter Eleven: Against All Odds — 195

Part Four: UNSTOPPABLE Future
Chapter Twelve: Believe — 215

Conclusion — 223
Resources — 227
Notes — 231

The following people have contributed to the creation of this book:

ADVOCATES
Pamm Larry
Dr. Vandana Shiva
Jeffrey Smith
Tami Canal
Robert F. Kennedy, Jr.
Vani Hari

HEALTH CARE PROVIDERS
Jill C. Carnahan, MD, ABFM, ABHM, IFMCP
Sarah Cusack, MPT, CHHC
Joel Kahn, MD
Jennifer Giustra-Kozek, LPC, NBCC, HpN

SCIENTISTS
Stephanie Seneff, Ph.D.
Gilles-Éric Séralini, Ph.D.
Michael Antoniou, Ph.D.
Michael Hansen, Ph.D.
Evaggelos Vallianatos, Ph.D.
Anthony Samsel, Ph.D.

MOM CONTRIBUTORS
Joanie
Vicki J.
Holly
Karen L.
Cindy S.
Karen Thomas
Julie J.
Belinda M.
Karina O.
Amberle M.
Cindy B.
Colleen G.
Margaret D.
Colleen C.
Rhonda L.
Laurie Olson
Susan Patterson

TEACHER
Julie K.

JOURNALIST
Carey Gillam

FARMERS
Bob Streit, Ph.D.
Howard Vlieger
Pat Trask
Ib Pedersen
Don Huber, Ph.D.
Michael McNeill, Ph.D.

FOREWORD

As a functional medicine doctor, I've seen firsthand the increase in chronic conditions in this country. Allergies, autism, autoimmune disease, cancer, obesity, and diabetes are undeniably on the rise. So much of what's causing this phenomenon is the sheer number of chemicals we are exposed to on a daily basis. In fact, I see environmental toxicity as the elephant in the room—the number one factor contributing to chronic disease.

Many doctors don't acknowledge the overwhelming evidence that we are exposed to an unprecedented number of chemicals—which are certainly impacting our health as a society. I see this as a twofold problem. First, medical students aren't taught about toxicity in terms of low-level accumulation over time. Second, many of these exposures are occurring so slowly and are even multigenerational, beginning in utero. The result is that it's taking the medical community decades to fully realize the impact of these chemicals on the human body.

Though the shift in the medical community appears to be slow, I see massive strides being made through functional medicine and through individuals taking the power of information and using it to control their personal health.

The massive increase in incidents of chronic conditions that have been caused in large part by a toxin burden has made the number one recommendation that I give to my patients to incorporate an organic, toxin-free lifestyle as much as humanly possible (and while keeping their sanity). I believe that the future of medicine must continue to rely heavily on people making comprehensive lifestyle changes. Ultimately, an individual can move more quickly and with purpose to bring about change than the major corporations that are the suppliers of these chemicals. However, as more individuals make the right choices, we can collectively force these giants to change, too.

We live in a time when it isn't safe to blindly eat something simply because it came from the grocery store. As a country, we are consuming mutant food whose production is completely under the control of money-driven corporations. Yet, I see a future where people can claim back the power over their bodies and health by taking matters into their own hands. Only through leveraging the accessibility of information can we fight against the onslaught of chemicals that are making us sick—and this is exactly what Zen Honeycutt's book *UNSTOPPABLE* does.

Her story begins as an exasperated mother of children who have relentless allergies and other health conditions. Her personal research, which was initially fueled out of fear for her children's lives, turns into an informed and calculated attack on the corporations that are making us sick.

She clearly outlines how our bodies are bombarded with tens of thousands of chemicals every single day. Her discussion includes how over eighty thousand chemicals have been approved by the Environmental Protection Agency since the 1940s, and a shocking majority of these chemicals are being added directly to our food with little or no oversight.

As it stands now, many of these chemicals are labeled "generally recognized as safe" by the Food and Drug Administration and remain in our food until enough people get sick. Though we are coming to realize that indeed much of the country is becoming sick due to our food system, many government agencies that regulate that food continue to turn a blind eye. Zen discovers this directly after testing breast milk for glyphosate—a powerful herbicide.

We've obviously become the guinea pigs for corporations such as Monsanto, an agrochemical and agricultural biotechnology corporation, and the government agencies put in place to protect us simply aren't doing their jobs. Fortunately, we live in a time when an impassioned mother can spread quality information and create influential groups such as Moms Across America, as Zen Honeycutt has done.

Personally, I grew up on a corn and soybean farm in central Illinois with massive exposure to pesticides—glyphosate, atrazine, and other organophosphates. Fortunately, my brothers have switched to 100 percent non-GMO farming with some organic farms, but this was not the case when I was growing up. My parents simply didn't have access to the information available today or the ability to easily transition the farm over. I've often wondered how many of my past personal health problems were due to the chemical exposure I grew up with. These chemicals must be taken seriously, and Zen's book is part of the light that needs to be shined on both how widespread and how sickening these chemicals actually are.

Foreword

Every day in my practice, I meet with mothers and their children who are baffled by the bizarre and chronic health conditions that are impacting their lives. After their first appointment with me, they are shocked that the information surrounding the state of our country's toxic food supply isn't common knowledge. Educating people about the importance of food in the country has changed dramatically over the last few decades, and Zen's book is one that captures the details of this seismic shift.

As Zen says, "A worried mom does better research than the FBI," and I have to say that when it comes to Zen's relentless pursuit of the truth, I have to agree. *UNSTOPPABLE* is backed with scientific research woven with Zen's own personal journey in a way that you'll relate and make you ready to join the fight. She takes terrifying situations and stares them down bravely—and frankly, that's what this country needs more of.

I believe that we are powerful and that we can stop the toxic food system from destroying our lives. We just need to educate ourselves and band together. The information in the book is critical to every single American's life—including yours.

Zen doesn't write to evoke groundless fears—she writes with the intention of awakening undeniable truths so that we may cause change. Change that future generations depend upon.

—JILL C. CARNAHAN, MD, ABFM, ABIHM, IFMCP

ACKNOWLEDGMENTS

ONE OF MY favorite things to do in this world is to acknowledge people. When I am a present witness to the love, energy, generosity, and uniqueness of that person, to me that is the essence of a fulfilling life. It is with great pleasure that I first acknowledge my husband Todd, who supported the tumultuous last five years during the growth of Moms Across America. Your generosity, humor, and faith in our mission kept me going.

I thank my son Ben for being intuitive, compassionate, and for inspiring me to be a speaker. I thank Bodee for inspiring me with his positive attitude and awesome determination to get better. I thank Bronson for bringing wonder and magic into our lives. I also thank my parents Mavis and Paul for being incredibly awe-inspiring sources of trust, faith, and encouragement. My brother Tao, my sister-in-law Amy, and my sister Chi have always listened to me share volumes of information with open-mindedness and grace. I cannot thank you enough for being supportive of my journey and of this cause.

I acknowledge the dedication and support of my selfless board. Laurie Olson, president, Natalie Paffrath, treasurer, and Judy Blake, former secretary, who bring sound decision-making and unique perspectives to the table that have allowed Moms Across America, and me, to grow in ways I never imagined.

I cannot say enough about Anne Temple, who has been my graphic designing guru, right hand, and source of endless amusement for years. She gets me through it all.

I wish to thank George Klabin who supports not only our work, but also a pathway to sustainability, being focused, and authentic. His encouragement, wisdom, and support give me faith in humanity.

Thank you to team members Esther Grondahl, Kat Furey, Kathy Borthwick, and Alex Carillo, and regional leaders of Moms Across America: Lisa Almendarez-Guermo, Amber King, Nanette Reetz, Jessica Denning, Illana Stern, Marcey Goetz-Than, Kathy Blum, Ellie Kirchner, Marghi Barnes, and Happel Kolokowski. Their commitment is changing our country.

I also thank the sponsors of Moms Across America—foundations, organizations, companies, and hundreds of individual donors who made everything in this book possible. I thank the volunteers and leaders who inspired me to take that tentative first step into activism: Dr. Vandana Shiva, Diana Reeves, Kerne Erickson, Paula Fitz, John Diaz, Pamm Larry, Bob McFarland, Kathleen Hallal, Robyn O'Brien, Rachel Linden, Arianne Glazer, and Jeffrey Smith.

I thank especially the farmer educators, who are leading the way: Howard Vlieger, Dr. Don Huber, John Kempf, Dr. Bob Streit, and Michael McNeill. I thank the doctors who are pioneering new pathways amid the mess of this food system: Dr. Matt Buckley, Dr. Zach Bush, Dr. Jill Carnahan, Dr. Ben Edwards, Dr. Joel Kahn, and Dr. Michelle Perro. Thank you to the lawyers from Richman Law Group and Miller Law Firm: Baum, Hedlund, Aristei, and Goldman, and Robert F. Kennedy, Jr.

I thank the coaches and leadership of Landmark, a personal training and development program that gave me the tools and distinctions to create many of the breakthroughs in my life that are described in this book.

It is with immense gratitude that I acknowledge the tremendous support and wisdom of my editor Debbie Luican. Her skill, grace, and dedication have made this experience one of the biggest blessings of my life. Debbie: this is your baby, too. Thank you.

There are literally hundreds of amazing people and organizations that have contributed immensely to the journey of creating this book and contributing to the impact of Moms Across America in the world. My only regret is that not all your names fit between these pages. If I have failed to include your name, please forgive me and know that I cherish the contribution you have made in my life and in the lives of millions of others through your support of our mission to create healthy communities.

INTRODUCTION
Things Have Changed

"If all the moms in the world knew how awesome they are, all the problems in the world would be fixed."

—KID PRESIDENT, YOUTUBE SENSATION

IN THE 1970S and 80s, when we had company for dinner, my mom would cook up an array of dishes . . . bright-green broccoli and thinly sliced beef with oyster sauce, golden curry chicken with potatoes, or savory garlic shrimp and snow peas. When she brought the dishes, steaming hot, to the table, one after another, she would smile and present them like they were gifts from her heart. When we didn't have company, simple meals like roast beef on toast, sloppy joes, or humble Chinese rice porridge called jook were still presented as the most wonderful meal ever. When she made new dishes, she would enjoy the food so much, closing her eyes and saying "Mmm mmm!" that we had to take a taste just to see what the fuss was all about.

Her meals were clearly an unspoken act of love and joy. We knew that she loved us because of how well she fed us, how much she enjoyed cooking for us, how colorful the dishes were, and how happy she was to present them to us and to see us eat and enjoy them.

We never once thought about whether or not the food was genetically modified, pesticide-free, organic, gluten-free, dairy-free, nut-free, dye-free, preservative-free, vegan, vegetarian, Paleo, or ketogenic.

As a family, we didn't have allergies, rashes, autism, autoimmune disease, asthma, nonalcoholic fatty liver disease, cancer, Crohn's disease, colitis, or Hashimoto's disease. We didn't even know anyone with those health issues.

We didn't know that food could be dangerous.

We weren't in a health crisis as a country.

Things have changed.

Today, millions of us Americans are struggling with sick family members. We are confused, tired, irritable, and often feel very lonely in our struggle. If you are sick, if your kids are sick, and Western medicine has offered no hope—you're not alone, and it's not too late. There are things that your doctor may not know and that big business and the government don't want you to know. My doctor didn't know why my son had life-threatening allergies. My mother didn't know. None of my friends knew why their family member was sick. And the problem was that we didn't know what we didn't know. Most people still don't. And the corporations that make the chemicals that are making us sick want to keep it that way. That's why they fight labeling, accountability, and hire lobbyists to persuade policy makers to look the other way. The concept, "What you don't know won't hurt you," is not only untrue, it is hurting us physically as well as destroying the trustability and structure of our government and the fabric of our society. The impact of toxic chemicals and the corruption of our government have created an epidemic of health issues that could bankrupt our nation. Toxic chemicals contribute to mental illness, increasing acts of violence, addictions, and more—which, in turn, threaten the security of our communities and our freedom as citizens. America and its citizens are in distress—and it's time for us to restore our health, security, prosperity, and future.

What most people don't know is that independent science now shows that seemingly unrelated health issues such as autism, allergies, autoimmune disease, infertility, mental illness, colitis, liver disease, and cancer are all related. They all stem from an unprecedented toxic burden.

The problem is that by the time you take your child to the doctor for help due to symptoms of toxic burden, the doctors can only try to manage the illness or symptoms in front of them—preventing the toxic burden from happening is no longer an option.

In this book, you will gain insights, information, tips, and inspiration to have a whole new life experience around food and health. It may feel like a switch has suddenly been turned on or that you have suddenly seen the light at the end of the tunnel. It may also feel threatening at first. But when you come to understand the effects of our food through my eyes, a struggling mom who had had enough and got down to business and decided to do something about it, it makes sense that our food is making us sick. You will be educated and moved by the contributions from a vast community of experts and other caring people. I will be real about the ups and downs and share with you what many people in America still do not know about food, toxins, and our health. I will share with you what I know, to my core, without a doubt, without a moment of wavering—that when moms are empowered, we can change the world. When people are empowered, when we truly get how awesome we are, we can transform entire systems, economies, education, governments, and the future. We are UNSTOPPABLE.

UNSTOPPABLE

PART ONE

UNSTOPPABLE LOVE

CHAPTER ONE
LOVE IN ACTION

"Being deeply loved by someone gives you strength, while loving someone deeply gives you courage."
—LAO TZU

TODAY, ALL OF us love someone who is sick. One out of two children in America has a chronic illness. One out of two males and one out of three females are expected to get cancer. One out of five has a mental illness, and one out of six has a learning disorder. One out of ten has nonalcoholic fatty liver disease . . . I could go on and on. Although the challenges of our health crisis are great, I have seen firsthand that the love for our families is greater. That love is driving a movement to transform our food supply, reduce its toxic burden, instill integrity in the regulatory agencies, and restore health in America.

Let's start at the beginning. I did not take it for granted that my husband and I would have children. After the tragedy of September 11, my mother used a travel credit to take my brother Tao, sister Chi, and I to Hawai'i to regroup. During that time, while my husband, Todd, and I were apart, I suggested to him that we each think about whether or not we really wanted to have children. One night in Waikiki I had a dream in which the face of a baby with curly black hair appeared. I felt it was a boy, and he said without moving his lips, "Let me be."

I had my first son, Ben, and then my second, Bodee (my only curly-haired baby), and then my third, Bronson, over the course of the next five years. Each time you have a child, your life changes drastically. It opens up in new ways. New problems, new solutions, new ways of eating, sleeping, and even breathing are foisted upon you. If your child is born or grows to be less than perfectly healthy, you suddenly have new feelings of fear and insecurity that you never could have imagined. Doubts set in. Parents find themselves disempowered by their children's persistent health issues. It impacts their relationships, marriages, effectiveness, and our society as a whole. So what can we do?

We try to cope. We redefine "normal," since nothing about our lives is the same as it was before. We are uncomfortable when we take solace in the fact that almost every kid on the block has multiple health issues—not only our children. We try to find relief in the fact that it may not be our fault . . . but that doesn't stop us from trying to find the reasons behind the health problems and the solutions to them, and to share them with our community. In our quest to redefine what it means to be healthy, we research, try new things, and persevere. What we ultimately end up redefining is ourselves.

In the first few months of motherhood, I was not the dewy-faced picture of happiness we often think we will be as parents. I was more of a bedraggled, anxious, incoherent mess. If you had a baby recently—or forty years ago—I am sure you remember the bleary-eyed haze of the first few months of your first child. Some moms are joyous like never before, easily breastfeeding or naturally co-sleeping. Others of us struggle with breastfeeding, need to bottle-feed, and feel guilty and exhausted. Others have postpartum depression. No matter what our childbirth or newborn baby experiences are, we can all relate to the challenges and the love we feel for our children.

I recall feeling like a cow experiencing sleep torture. My son Ben nursed every two hours and he broke out in a rash nearly every time. He cried much more than I ever imagined possible. In my first week of being a new mom, a mother of eight, tried to soothe me by saying, "When you are a new mom, you feel like something is wrong 99 percent of the time when the reality is that everything is exactly perfect 99 percent of the time."

For the most part, her words set me at ease and allowed me to enjoy my son. But when his rashes persisted, his crying increased, and his poo turned bright green, and well . . . I won't go into any more details . . . I trusted my gut and took him to the doctor. It turned out that he had a milk allergy. I was truly forlorn. I gave up all dairy products and spent the first year and a half of his life gazing longingly at ice cream, pizza, and cheese and wondering why this had happened to my child.

I never had a milk allergy, or any other allergy, when I was a child and neither did my husband, Todd. But as I spoke to other new moms in our moms club, I realized that many of us had babies with allergies to milk and soy. None of us knew why. We all thought there must be some genetic predisposition for our children to be this way even though there was no reason to think so. We did not admit it, but deep down, we blamed ourselves and struggled, wondering, *Did I do something wrong?* Was it something I ate while pregnant? Did inducing him with Pitocin to be born when he perhaps was not "ready" alter his immune system? Was it the epidural they gave me during labor? My unanswered questions fell on deaf ears at the doctor's office and my mom friends and I would commiserate in our joint confusion. But we powered on.

When Ben was four months old, shortly after I had stopped drinking milk or eating cheese, and when I felt like I was at my wit's end the night before Mother's Day, my son slept through the night for the first time. For eight hours. That same night, I had a dream. He was in his co-sleeper bassinet and he looked at me. Ben spoke to me and said, "Thank you, Mom. I love you." The connection a mother feels with her child is beyond science, beyond explanation, and it is very real.

I woke up filled with joy. I was rested and fulfilled. It was the most wonderful Mother's Day, and what Ben had said to me in the dream was the most wonderful gift he could have given me. Sometimes, all we need, as mothers, is a moment of reprieve so that we can be grateful for the opportunity before us. I knew then that I would do anything for my son—even if being tired was part of the deal.

In the first months of our children's lives, we refocus and see what truly matters to us. My breastfeeding lactation consultant looked me in the eyes when I was worn out from cracked nipples and breastfeeding struggles and told me, "Your *only job* for the first three months of his life is to feed him, eat, and sleep."

Her words released a sigh from deep within my clenched chest that I had been holding on to for weeks. I let go of all the "to do's" on my list. I shifted how I saw my world and allowed myself to "just" be a mom. She gave me the freedom to power on, with focus.

"You don't need to do *anything* else," she reminded me as we parted. "You do not need to have people over, do the dishes, or clean the house. Let someone else do that."

If I didn't hug and kiss her it was only because I was successfully nursing my baby at that moment. Todd wanted me to be happy. He willingly stepped up and did the dishes and took care of everything. My mom came to visit, and I allowed her to help. It was challenging to watch them doing things differently than I would have, but I let it go.

No matter where you are in the stages of being a mom, a woman, and a human being . . . look at what you are struggling with.

> Is the situation beyond your current understanding or ability to cope? Usually, if you are struggling, there is simply something you are not aware of yet that will help you overcome the obstacle.
>
> 1. **Ask for help.** Bring in the experts—someone who has personally experienced and mastered that area. Listen, be open, and try what they suggest.
>
> 2. **Be willing to let go of your original plan.** So what if the house is not cleaned today, you can't make mac-n-cheese as you normally do for a potluck, or your project is not turning out? Things change. Breathe. Let go.
>
> 3. **Be willing to accept help**—and again, **be willing for everything to not go according to your plan** when other people help you. Be okay with the fact that others will do things differently than you do. It's okay. Really.

The Erosion of Health and Mom Power

As soon as Ben began to tolerate milk occasionally, at around eighteen months old, he developed a new allergy.

"It's just a rash," people said over and over. "Relax. It will go away." But my mother's intuition was telling me different.

It did of course, eventually, go away . . . but not before serious doubt had set in. Why did he rash out all over his body? What did we do? Was it the dog, or the walnuts my mother had given him? Why did she give him a nut at twenty-two months old? Why didn't she know better?

Wait . . . why should she "know better"? What's wrong with nuts? Haven't humans been eating nuts for all of recorded history? Why, suddenly, are there so many kids with nut allergies? Why don't I know this? And these questions were followed by the inevitable, "What did I do wrong?"

I had taken Ben to all his scheduled doctor visits. I fed him healthy food, used body care products without parabens, and we lived in an area with fairly clean air. And yet, still, I must have done something wrong.

Health issues in our children erode not only our sense of safety but also confidence in ourselves as caretakers.

My brain reeled with questions, and I found myself researching an endless loop of illnesses: autoimmune diseases, eczema, psoriasis, and allergies. Dairy, soy, and nuts were at the top of the list for most common childhood allergens. One friend of mine had Celiac disease, and another was gluten intolerant. I had never heard of these conditions as a child, so I had chalked them up as extreme cases. These people just had bad luck. *My son didn't have those problems and never would,* I thought to myself. *He's a healthy kid!*

I think to protect my own self-image as a mother, I chose to be resigned to and doubtful about my son's allergies. I chose to see the situation as our new normal. He got rashes now and then. That was that.

When the rashes became practically a weekly occurrence, however, I could no longer accept it as normal. I took him to the allergist that my doctor had recommended, and he told me he needed to do a series of sixty skin prick tests, with needles. I cringed and folded into my own lap, holding my face in my hands. My heart hurt for Ben's impending pain. I knew from our experience with vaccinating (which I now regret) that he would scream holy hell and my guilt would be unbearable. So, when we got home, I quietly asked my husband to take him back for the skin prick tests.

> Consider that it does not always *have to* be you doing everything and you do not have to feel guilty if you don't. In fact, thinking that you do is disempowering. *"Have to" equals stress. There is no "have to," there is only choice.* In some cases, letting go and allowing others to care for your child can empower everyone.

He agreed. When he came home the first time he said it was miserable. The second time was just torture. I have no idea how he got my son to co-operate the second time, once Ben knew what was going to happen. I can only say I am glad I was not there. Todd, however, was a rock . . . until he came home. Then he lost it. It was not okay for his son to be sick. He was angry. But he also realized how much he loved his son. That was a bonding moment for them. I think it was the first time that my husband felt solely responsible for his child's care in a time of distress. His fatherly instincts kicked in, and he got interested in our son's health issues. He became very attentive and protective from that moment on and they now have a very close bond. I learned that giving my husband an opportunity to take on challenging situations with our son allowed them to create a stronger relationship. I have since released the guilt I had about letting my son go through some tough things without me. I don't have to "do it all" after all—and sometimes it's better if I don't.

The test came back showing Ben had allergies to dozens of things: tomatoes, grasses, trees, mushrooms, dogs, and walnuts . . . some mild, and some off the charts. The results told me that I was going to have to increase my efforts in how I managed the frequency and severity of the rashes. The doctor gave no indication whatsoever that my son would ever actually be completely well. In fact, he warned that nut allergies often get worse with every exposure and can become life-threatening. I was convinced that there was something "wrong" with Ben's immune system and that was just the way it was. He was more sensitive. We needed to be extra careful. Period.

His walnut allergy rated in the life-threatening category—a nineteen on a scale with a high of twenty—and extended into a tree nut allergy. His body later proved this on Thanksgiving night.

Thanksgiving Dinner

One minute we were sitting at a huge table of happy relatives, all stuffing our faces with turkey and cranberry sauce—and the next minute my five-year-old son Ben was looking at me with a pleading in his eyes that spoke of misery.

I asked Ben what the matter was and if he was okay. When he said his stomach hurt, I told him to go to the guest room and lay down. I thought that he must be coming down with a bug and should rest.

Moments later, though, he cried out from the back room and my husband and I ran to him. He was covered from head to toe in large, raspberry-like bumps. He was swollen and red. What was happening? I had a sudden realization. Nuts. I wanted to scream, but it came out a fierce whisper. *"Nothing he ate had nuts in it, did it?"*

We had specifically asked my mother-in-law to tell everyone not to bring food with nuts. My mother-in-law and father-in-law consulted with each other and a few cousins and figured out that there were pecans in the stuffing.

That cousin had not gotten the email or message. She always made her stuffing that way. I had not asked. I had served it to my son.

Thank God, we had filled the prescription for the EpiPen and I had it in my purse. I couldn't bear to use it, so my husband did. He jammed the needle into my son's thigh and we both gasped as Ben screamed in pain. When the EpiPen seemed "stuck" in his leg I went to pull it out, yanked it, and blood spurted out of the wound in an arc for several feet. My mother-in-law cried out, I felt sick, and my husband swooped Ben into his arms and began carrying him to the door to rush him to the hospital. I tried to apply pressure to the wound as we ran. We did not even think of waiting for an ambulance. There was no way we could wait—we had to move.

As I buckled my son into his car seat I noticed that his eyes were glazing over. Then his eyeballs rolled back in his head and I pleaded with him, "Stay with us, Ben! You can do it! Breathe!"

His head drooped, and his body became limp. My head felt light, and shapes around me blurred as I realized my child could die. He moaned in pain. I rubbed his chest and talked to him as much as I could. The fear was choking me. My husband drove as fast as he could to the nearest hospital and they let us in immediately.

We were ushered directly to a bed in the ER. They were stony-faced as they told us to lay him down and step back. They didn't ask any questions after we told him that he had a nut allergy and had eaten a nut, they behaved as if this were a routine incident.

The nurses moved like silent robots as they injected him with steroids and an IV. I held his hand and prayed to God. Once the steroids kicked in, he opened his eyes and looked at me with that pleading look that said to me, "Help me," I just kept saying, "It's okay, it's okay, you are going to be okay. I love you, Sweetie. Daddy loves you. We are right here." But what I really felt was helpless. My son lay swollen, bumpy, and in critical condition for hours. There was nothing I could do but pray.

I know now that a few minutes more and we could have lost him. The swelling of his body could have closed his airways and within minutes he would have been unable to breathe. We would not have been able to resuscitate him on our own—he would have needed a tube. There are hundreds of parents who lose their child from nut allergies every year—even with an EpiPen or even with a doctor as a parent. It just so happened that we made it to the hospital in time that night.

When we left the hospital with him, and monitored his recovery at home, it began to sink in that our son had almost died from Thanksgiving dinner, from food. I grappled with this concept with the tenacity of a mother tiger tracking her enemy. I asked my husband repeatedly, "How did this happen? Why is he allergic? Why did he almost die from food? What are we going to do about this? What if he eats a cookie at a friend's house and we are not there?" As if he could actually answer me.

He did the best he could by saying, "We just have to be really careful. He cannot eat nuts. We don't have them in our house. We double-check everything he eats, and he just doesn't eat at friends' houses. There is nothing else we can do. We do the best we can."

I didn't like it. It wasn't enough for me. I wanted reassurance that this would never happen again. What if we went to a friend's house and he grabbed a cookie while the family was watching a movie? Asphyxiation is silent. The voices in my head were not only disempowering, they were downright disastrous. Suddenly, every committee member of doom was hollering in my head how tree nuts were going to infiltrate our lives and cause a severe allergic reaction in my son.

The hospital doctor had confirmed my fears by warning us that "children do not usually grow out of nut allergies." He said that "every exposure to nuts increases the severity of the next allergic reaction," so the next one "could be fatal." I felt completely justified in increasing the severity of my anxiety. My sense of being capable of caring for my son and keeping him safe was eroding. I was a mom in survival mode. I was just doing what needed to be done to keep him alive.

Playdates became minefields of peanut butter crackers and chocolate chip cookies that could have hidden walnuts. Friends' houses became places where rather than feeling relaxed and at ease, grateful to be in a space that I didn't have to clean myself, I felt on guard and uncomfortable. There could be a bowl of nuts on the coffee table or Nutella on the sticky hands of their toddler.

It may not seem like a "big deal" to anyone else for someone to have a child with a nut or food allergy—after all, "it's just a rash" and it will go away . . . but the fact is that a mom of a child with a life-threatening nut or food allergy is suddenly the mom of a child whose life is threatened . . . *all* . . . *the* . . . *time*. Especially when they eat—which seems to be all the time. Sharing a meal is the time when a mom usually is able to express her love through food. My mom would beam when saw us happily eating the meal she prepared us. Mealtime is when families celebrate tradition and special occasions with food. It is a time to relax, indulge, and enjoy. Not for a mom of a child with food allergies, however. She is on guard. She is seriously analyzing the surroundings and protecting her child. *Food is no longer fun. Other people's food is not a treat—it is a threat.*

> If you are stressed out and angry and don't know why, consider that having loved ones be threatened by serious health issues is a pretty darn good reason. Give yourself a break. Be gentle with yourself. Give yourself space and time to deal with your feelings.
>
> If you meet people at parties or at school and they don't seem very warm or happy, or if they seem stressed and angry, don't take it personally and don't be offended or judge them. Be compassionate. Know that they could have a family member in the hospital or have just lost their sister to breast cancer. More often than not, this is the case. People are stressed out today. We need to be the people who will listen, support, and care.

Anything Is Possible . . . the Open Door to Discovery

The social structure for modern families is not in a woman's best interest. Transplants with no grandma, mother, aunt, or sister nearby to support us as new mothers, we are often left alone, exhausted, resentful, and fearful. I was grateful to have one good friend with a baby my son's age and a small group of La Leche League moms to turn to for support. Still, I felt stressed. I didn't think that I could have another child and handle even more stress, but I didn't want my first child to be lonely, and I knew the value of siblings. So, we were fortunate to conceive again. Bodee was also born in a hospital. Just as with my first delivery (both births were natural, so the babies got the full dose of good bacteria and microbes that come from that process to support their immune system), I was also pumped full of Pitocin—even though my water broke naturally. I also had an epidural, which numbed all my senses. Bodee arrived a healthy eight pounds with a full head of curly hair. I had gained sixty pounds during that pregnancy. I thought this was normal.

Bodee was happy, alert, and challenging. He often tested my patience by doing things like snatching a Costco five-pound bag of shredded cheddar cheese, dumping it on his carpeted bedroom floor, rolling in it, and cackling with glee. His M.O. was to have fun. He delighted in winning games, being first, and later, being a straight A student.

Bodee was healthy and did not exhibit any health issues for years. What I began to notice was that my own health was suffering.

Put the Oxygen Mask on Yourself First...

"Your children do not grow up to treat themselves the way you treated them, they grow up to treat themselves the way you treated yourself."
—OPRAH WINFREY

One day, I realized I needed to nap every day for two hours. Since my youngest at the time was well past nursing and not waking me up anymore during the night, I could not blame my children's sleep habits for my fatigue. Something was wrong. A healthy thirty-four-year-old woman doesn't nap every day. I was irritable and foggy after meals, snapping at my loved ones or retreating and being antisocial at parties. Since I had never had allergies as a child, I didn't even consider that allergies could be a possibility. I just thought my fatigue was hormonal.

It was around this time that I did the Landmark Forum, a personal training and development course that promises you will "live life fully and live a life you love." I wanted that. I had been angry, fearful, and stressed out for years. I wanted something different and I was willing to do something about it. In that class, and in subsequent courses with Landmark, I created remarkable breakthroughs in my life. The main lesson I learned, down to my bone marrow, was that anything is possible. Although this sounds idealistic and naive, it actually gave me power, responsibility, and integrity unlike anything I had ever seen before. My life today is beyond what I ever imagined, largely due to the tools I got at Landmark.

One day I got an email from an old friend about an iridologist—an alternative health practitioner who scans and analyzes the patterns, colors, and other characteristics of the iris to determine information about a patient's systemic health. I was inclined to reject the idea as woo woo medicine. But then I thought, since it worked so well for her . . . maybe the idea that "anything is possible" could apply here . . . and I wouldn't know unless I tried. So

I made an appointment with the iridologist/herbalist/naturopath, and was amazed at the results.

First, she could immediately tell by looking at my iris that I was intolerant to gluten and that dairy (I was eating it again) was causing a mucus build up in my body. She said I was grinding through the day, probably very tired and wanting to nap. This was something I had not told her—she just saw it in the iris scan. She also knew that I was anemic when I was seven years old. She could tell that I had experienced severe stress the same year that my parents got divorced. The irises in our eyes are like tree trunks, and the groves mark significant events in time. Lack of nutrients, stress, and illness are all recorded in the lines of the iris. Whether it was "woo woo" or not, I was willing to listen to her and give her advice a shot.

She told me to go gluten-free for six months and dairy-free for six weeks (dairy can increase mucus build up in the body, making it hard to cleanse). She had me do a parasite cleanse and take a few herbs and supplements that I bought from a local health food store.

I did *not* want to believe that I was gluten intolerant, but I was willing to try eliminating gluten from my diet because I had nothing to lose. Anything would be a step up from what I was feeling. When my husband and other family members doubted the diagnosis, I got a blood test from a Western medical doctor, and it did confirm I was intolerant to one protein in wheat—a new modern protein called gliadin. It was my worst nightmare, and one that millions of people in America face today.

One out of every four people (especially people with type O blood) over the age of thirty develops a gluten intolerance, and many don't know it. It's the cause of fatigue, weight gain that is almost impossible to reverse, fogginess (read mommy brain!), and irritability. Gluten intolerance can lead to depression and can even play a major role in contributing to schizophrenia.

I drank the psyllium husk cleanse she recommended every morning, went both gluten-free and dairy-free, and within two weeks I started feeling much better. Six weeks later, I felt like a new person. I was no longer napping—in fact, I was not even interested in a nap. I was sixteen pounds lighter, with a waistline that curved inward like a nineteen-year-old's! I bought a bikini! I was happier, more cheerful, and my head was clearer. The diet became a lifestyle change (except for occasional cheese) and I felt great.

I will admit it was difficult and sad at times. I truly mourned the loss of French bread, pizza at parties, and crackers with goat cheese at a friend's house. I mourned donuts, croissants, birthday cake, and pie. It was once inconceivable . . . but I didn't eat pie.

I maintained the shift in eating because I wanted to cleanse and heal my body. My cousin told me that she went gluten-free for a year and now she can eat gluten now and then. I wanted that. I did not want to be restricted forever . . . I wanted to be able to eventually eat a croissant again. I couldn't bear the idea of never again.

Later, when I became pregnant with my third boy, Bronson, and I ate gluten free, I only gained twenty-five pounds, versus the fifty and sixty pounds with my previous two pregnancies, and yet he was my biggest baby. I had watched *The Business of Being Born* movie, and this time gave birth at home, in the water, with a midwife, a doula, and my husband. It was one of the most empowering experience's of my life. Bronson's first word was "yes." My husband and I like to say we are creating a world of *yes*.

Today, because I have taken steps to heal my gut by eliminating nonorganic foods, adding fermented foods, and taking supplements to support gut health, I can tolerate small amounts of modern wheat. I can also enjoy normal portions of organic, ancient grains that do not contain any gliadin. If I eat the standard American diet, however, which includes a lot of nonorganic wheat, I feel foggy, cranky, and tired. It really is not worth it.

> Check in . . . Are you taking care of yourself?
> How do you feel after you eat conventional (nonorganic) wheat? Dairy? Are there certain foods that leave you not feeling your best?
> Eliminate these foods from your diet, and after two weeks, reintroduce them and see how you feel. You may notice that the tired, foggy, irritable feeling that you used to feel and just thought was "normal" is actually not normal, and those foods are not worth it.

More and More Allergies . . .

It wasn't long after I was comfortable being gluten-free that I began to notice the same changes in behavior in my eldest son, Ben, after he ate wheat. He got cranky, whiny, tired, and couldn't focus well. His grades dropped, and he began to hate school. He cried every morning about not wanting to go to school and had dark circles under his eyes. This time, instead of the allergist, I took him to the same iridologist and she confirmed a gluten allergy. I was devastated. To add to my struggle, the iridologist's assessment was not enough for my husband and family members. They did not want to believe it. I didn't argue with them. I just got his blood tested, which confirmed the iridologist's findings, and gave them the lab reports that showed he was gluten intolerant. Then I asked for their help. They agreed to give it.

Bodee also developed rashes when he was three years old, and I knew from experience to take him to the doctor right away. I immediately had his blood tested (I could not bear the pin prick tests) and learned, after years of his eating eggs almost every day, that he was suddenly allergic to eggs. All of my sons had most of their vaccinations. Vaccinations often have egg in them, along with a whole host of other ingredients that I did not know about at the time. I later learned, after Bronson developed a peanut allergy when he had never eaten peanuts, that some vaccines contain undisclosed peanut oil. It wasn't until years later that I read all of the ingredients in vaccines and began to suspect their involvement in my son's health issues.

Regardless of what I believe caused the food allergies, both of my sons had them. Lots of them. Bronson would puff up just being in a restaurant with peanut shells on the floor. We had to stop going to the traditional family favorite restaurant for his father's birthday. The food system was really beginning to piss me off. We had to manage multiple allergies with every meal. Egg, milk, and gluten/wheat allergies are very challenging, as those ingredients are in most of our American meals, sauces, and treats. I was exhausted by the thought of cooking. The world became a place of "no's." It was not fun.

Once again, I felt resigned that my children would just have to deal with their allergies and I was doubtful that anything would ever change.

The Mystery Deepened

For years, I struggled with multiple allergies in my children, not knowing why they had them. Doctors had no explanation. I was frustrated every day. I feared for my sons' futures. I began hearing how more and more friends of mine had children with soy, corn, dairy, and nut allergies. Then I started hearing of children with allergies to bananas, apples, and mangoes. I saw mothers of children with rare diseases on television talking about how their children were only able to eat six foods. The overwhelming response to that show made it clear that these conditions were not so rare. More and more children were allergic to very common foods such as pepper, parsley, fish, chicken, and watermelon. Who was allergic to watermelon? What was happening?

The growing allergies and health issues dominated the conversations at my moms' club. We were all worried and tense. I was definitely not empowered. When my eldest son, Ben, suddenly began displaying a new reaction—a red line around his mouth after eating, and lips that got swollen, inflamed, painful, and then flaky and dry after a week or so—I became increasingly anxious. He was eating a variety of foods, all of which we thought were healthy, so we could not pinpoint exactly which one was causing the reaction.

> Are you resigned? Are you *sure* that your child or family member has a disease, disorder, or condition that is incurable? Check in . . . how do you see this situation? Is it helpless? How do you see yourself in dealing with this situation? Are you hopeless? It's time to get authentic with yourself so you can take the next step.

Our Western medical doctors just prescribed different creams. They did not know the *reason* for this clown-mouth red rash. They said it was "contact dermatitis," but he wasn't touching anything to the outside of his mouth. It was not chapped lips. It looked like he had put a vacuum cleaner around his mouth. It was not a pleasant sight. He was extremely brave to go to school with that rash. I would have wanted to stay home and hide from the world.

After seven months of eliminating various foods, and on and off displays of the rash that lasted for one to two weeks each time, I was desperate. I gave up on the doctors and their creams and took him to the iridologist again. I had no idea what she would say. She took one look at him, scanned his iris, and pointed at the computer screen image of a few dots on his iris. "Oh, that's a carrageenan allergy."

"A caren-what-en?" I asked. This would be fun to explain to my mother-in-law . . . no Western medical doctor could prove this allergy with a blood test. It just wasn't an option.

"Carrageenan," she said again. "It's a seaweed food thickener they put in just about everything that kids like . . . hot dogs, ice cream, lunch meats, sauces, salad dressing, candy—even many organic foods and rice, soy and almond milk. You really have to read all the labels."

I wanted to cry. I wanted to throw my hands up in the air and quit.

I already had to navigate around wheat/gluten, dairy products, eggs, mushrooms, red food dye, tree nuts, and peanuts. I had just been able to get other family members on board. Now carrageenan, too? What the heck was I supposed to feed my kids? Birdseed? I went home defeated. It took me twice as long to grocery shop because I had to read every label, and our choices seemed to be fewer and fewer. I began to doubt her simply because I didn't want her diagnosis to be correct.

The information and the supplements the iridologist suggested helped the severity of the outbreaks, but they didn't help them go away completely, so I took him to a Chinese herbalist. She talked about yin and yang, and eating food that doesn't cause heat. I was too exhausted to pay much attention. I just wanted some kind of herbal medicine—a solution that would make the rash go away. She gave us a fine, brown powder mixture of herbs, that my son said tasted like nothing, to mix with warm water. Immediately, his rash did get better. It went completely away a few days later.

But then I fed him organic chicken lunch meat (thinking organic was less processed, so it would be healthier) and he instantly flared up again. I remembered that the iridologist had mentioned that carrageenan can be in lunch meat, so I looked at the package. Sure enough, in organic chicken lunch meat, there was carrageenan. Now I knew for sure that the iridologist was right. There was no Western medical doctor's test needed to back this one up and prove it to my husband and in-laws. This was it.

But why? Why could my son eat a hot dog or organic chicken sandwich one day, but not the next? What was going on with him? Or, perhaps more to the point, what was going on with the food?

I looked up carrageenan allergies online and found that, if left undiagnosed, such an allergy often led to stomach ulcers and stomach cancer. There were stories of children as young as twelve years old getting stomach cancer. Whoa. The *C* word. Not my child. Not on my watch.

The good news was I learned that a rash is the body's way of communicating that inflammation is going on in the gut. A lot of people think of a rash as a bad thing, but it's not. It's like the body's flashing red light—a warning. A rash is a good thing.

Too many people just slap a cream on a rash and hope it goes away. I was doing that, and it didn't work. The rash only develops into something else—often something painful. Your body communicates to you that something is wrong through pain signals. I did not want to wait until then.

I researched. I don't remember how I came upon Robyn O'Brien's TEDx Talk (I think someone shared it on Facebook), but that moment changed my life and my kids' lives forever.

It is important that we share our stories, as I have shared mine with you. It helps us to cope and opens up space for us to then create a new future.

- Have you ever told someone the nitty gritty of your story? Often, we keep our stories to ourselves to hide what we think of as inadequacies as a parent or spouse. Hiding these stories can cause more stress for our bodies. Share your story with a friend.

- At the same time, do not *become* your story. Don't let it define you or how others see you—say, as *a mom of sick kids*. That's not who you are, it's not the way you want to get attention, and it's not how you want your kids to know you as a parent, either. You also don't want your child to identify him or herself as a "sick kid." It's something you are both dealing with and getting support in transitioning out of.

- Don't compare. If my story is not nearly "as bad" as yours, or if my story is something you have never experienced, don't get caught in the trap of comparing. Comparison can become a crutch for justifying why you cannot do anything. For example: *My situation is much worse and therefore impossible to change . . .* or, *We're fine—we aren't dealing with food allergies, so we don't need to look at what we are eating . . .*

Just look at your situation. If you are struggling with anything, at any level, that is not working for you, now is the time to be honest with yourself.

CHAPTER TWO

LEARNING THE TRUTH ABOUT GMOS

"I always wondered why somebody doesn't do something about that, then I realized I was somebody."
—LILY TOMLIN

THE LOVE FOR my child led me to research things I had never considered. My moment of discovery about GMOs (genetically modified organisms) lead me to a whole new understanding of the food system, our government, and how the world works. Robyn O'Brien's TEDx Talk introduced a completely foreign concept to me in an unthreatening way. This is why it had tens of thousands of views at the time and over a million today. When her child puffed up as a result of eating food she began to wonder, "Why is my child allergic to food? What is a food allergy?" She learned it was when the body detected a foreign invader. Then she asked whether there were foreign invaders in our food. She discovered that the answer was yes. In 1996, food manufacturers introduced milk with genetically modified growth hormone, and soy and corn that were also GMO.

The Codex Alimentarius Commission (CODEX) is an intergovernmental body with over one hundred and eighty members established by the Food and Agriculture Organization (FAO) of the United Nations and the World Health Organization (WHO). CODEX defines genetically modified (GM) foods as foods derived from organisms whose genetic material (DNA) has been modified in a way that does not occur naturally, one example is the introduction of a gene from a different organism. Most GMOs in the food supply have the DNA of one species injected into the DNA of another species, creating a foreign protein. Newer GMOs have DNA or RNA which is edited and has been shown to cause mutations within the species.

Robyn wondered if foreign protein had something to do with her child's allergies. She then went on to describe all the health issues that have skyrocketed since GMOs were put in our food. She also explained that sixty-two (the data is now sixty-four) other countries label and twenty-four ban GMOs, but not the United States. My blood began to boil. She said that our food manufacturers such as Kraft, General Mills, and Kellogg's make non-GMO cereals for Europe and Asia, but *not* for the USA! What? Why? Because we are too naive to demand it? Why isn't the media telling us about GMOs? Why did the government allow GMOs in the first place?

I felt deep betrayal squeeze my heart. I was in a dark place. I did not want to believe that my government could not be trusted, but I realized it was true. Everything that Robyn said made sense. Her realization, explained in an easy to understand, relatable manner, shook me to my core.

I felt alone, unsafe, and depressed. I watched Robyn's TEDx Talk at least three times and then I began my search for more information. Robyn described herself as a "reluctant crusader." Like Robyn, initially I didn't want to be an activist. But the more I learned about GMOs and chemical farming, the less reluctant I became. Soon, I didn't want just the information. I didn't want to just understand the problem or learn how to cope with the problem. I wanted to *solve* the problem. I wanted the problem to not exist in the first place. I wanted to transform our food supply. I realized immediately that to achieve such a goal I couldn't be a reluctant activist—I needed to be part of an enthusiastic team. Even more, I needed a committed contingency for the long haul.

I didn't want to have to fight for something—I wanted to create a safe future for my children. Over time, I came to understand that this was not a war—it was an undertaking of community awakening and empowerment. I wanted to launch a campaign to create a new future. I needed input and support from scientists, doctors, farmers, journalists, politicians, and the moms who were finding solutions every day. We all needed to come together, each offering our unique understanding of the problems and potential solutions for bringing good health back to this country.

Transforming the food supply would take strategy, passion, courage, and leadership. The first step was to be a leader for my family's food choices and for their health. I resolved to be the one to make the change for my family. I would research and then find a way to convince my family to change our eating habits. Then I would take on the food supply.

At first, I had no idea how much I had to learn, and how discriminating I would have to become about the sources of the information I trusted. When I started digging, I soon realized that every one of my sources had to be questioned, and my information should come from a diverse community—not just a few scientists with links to big chemical companies that funded their research. Learning information, sourced from a vast number of different types of people from different communities, became a full-time job for me. My wish is that, with this book, you can build your foundation of knowledge and empowerment in a much shorter period of time.

Understanding the Problem

I learned from a Facebook post about the movie *Genetic Roulette* and that it was showing for free in July of 2012. I watched it immediately. I was aghast. Jeffrey M. Smith had been researching GMOs for seventeen years. He was not a scientist, but he could communicate the science because he had been interviewing scientists and doctors for nearly two decades. His description of GMOs went into great detail and showed, category by category, how GMOs were likely the cause of or a major contributing factor to allergies, autism, autoimmune diseases, miscarriages, and birth defects. At this stage in the food movement, almost everyone was focused on the dangers of GMOs and not the related pesticides, including me. Because GMOs were new at the time, and pesticides were commonly perceived to be harmless and able to be washed off, the food movement focused solely on GMOs.

> *Years ago, people told me that they could tell the difference when they ate GMOs versus non-GMOs. Frankly, I didn't believe them. For some reason, I thought the detrimental effects would be too slow and subtle for an individual to notice. But once I spoke with physicians who had prescribed non-GMO diets to thousands of patients, and even visited their clinics to speak with the patients firsthand, I realized just how quickly—and dramatically—people can respond. For some, chronic conditions disappeared in just days or weeks.*
>
> *I then asked audience members at more than 150 lectures to share their health improvements after they switched to non-GMO diets (or to share their patients' responses, if I was addressing a medical conference). The results were consistent. When the Institute for*

Responsible Technologysurveyed their subscribers, 3,256 responders reported the same thing.

We can say with confidence that there are now thousands of people who report significant health improvements in a range of conditions when they remove GMOs. This is confirmed by numerous health-care practitioners who prescribe non-GMO diets and see the same type of recoveries. When livestock and pets are taken off GMOs, vets and animal owners report similar improvements. And lab animals fed GMOs or Roundup suffer from these types of conditions.

Moreover, if we look at the side effects of the GMO process and the characteristics of Bt toxin and Roundup (both found in GMOs), we can understand why these particular conditions may be caused or exacerbated by eating GMOs. It is no surprise that the types of conditions linked to eating GMOs are rising in the U.S. population—closely correlated with the increased use of GMOs and Roundup.

—JEFFREY SMITH, founder of the
Institute for Responsible Technology, author, and
movie producer of *Genetic Roulette* and *Secret Ingredients*

Okay folks, we're going to get into the science for the next few pages. It's not easy but it's necessary. I suggest you power through, then come back and re-read it if you are moved to do so. This is complicated stuff and the chemical companies are hoping you'll just gloss over this information because the more of us who understand what is really going on in the food supply, the harder things are for Big Ag. But the more we know, the faster our food supply is transformed, and the healthier our families will be. So I am going to give it to you straight up.

GMOs have been highly contested, while proponents of GMOs say that they are safe. They say that GMOs happen in nature all the time—like a hybrid. However, GMOs are created only in a lab with a gene gun and by a process that scientists have patented to protect their technology. GMOs are not hybrids. Genetic engineering, for example, the altering of DNA with foreign species, or editing out DNA to remove a trait from a species permanently, does not happen naturally. It is not found in nature in any shape or form. The scientists and media that say GMOs are natural are misleading the public. Many of these scientists are not impartial, but are instead supported by advertising dollars or grants to universities from the GMO/chemical manufacturers and have incentives to make these claims. Regardless of their reasoning, they are certainly ignoring the "precautionary principle"—the principle that the introduction of a new product or process whose ultimate effects are disputed or unknown should be resisted. Any scientist worth his or her salt will admit that many aspects of GMOs are still unknown.

Here's what we do know—there are three general types of GMOs:

Bt Toxins

In a Bt (*Bacillus thuringiensis*) GMO corn, for instance, the Bt toxin from the carcass of a dead grain caterpillar is genetically engineered to *continuously* reproduce itself and create Bt toxin. It does not dry up and die off as it does naturally in organic farming practices. The GMO Bt toxin becomes a toxin factory. It is then put into the transfer "vehicle," so to speak, of the cauliflower mosaic virus or other bacteria and injected into the DNA of the corn so that every single cell of the plant becomes infected with this virus or bacteria with the Bt toxin factory inside. When the corn rootworm eats any part of the corn plant, the Bt toxin creates a toxin factory in the rootworm's stomach. The toxins cause holes in the worm's stomach that break open, the toxin leaks into the worm's body, and the rootworm dies. *Bt GMO corn is a registered pesticide with the EPA.* Most people would agree that a toxin that explodes the stomach of a bug is not a toxin that they would care to be eating in their corn chips, cereal, or tacos.

Herbicide Tolerant GMOs

Herbicide tolerant (HT) GMOs—typically corn, soy, sugar beets, canola, and cottonseed—are genetically engineered to resist herbicides, so farmers can drive a spraying tractor or aerial spray an entire field and kill only the weeds. Over 80 percent of the herbicide tolerant GMO crops have been engineered to withstand glyphosate herbicides. Glyphosate, originally used as a pipe cleaner, is the declared active chemical ingredient in Roundup. Hundreds of millions of pounds of glyphosate herbicides are used in the USA every year. Although proponents claim that GMOs are not significantly different from non-GMOs, new scientific studies show otherwise. There is more than one problem with GMO technology and glyphosate-tolerance traits:

1. Glyphosate herbicides do not dry off, wash off, or cook off. They are absorbed into the cells of the plant. The EPA has set "allowable" levels of glyphosate residue on about 160 of our food and feed crops between 0.2 and 400 parts per million (ppm), far higher than has been shown to cause harm. Obviously, we as human beings are not genetically engineered to resist herbicides. When we consume the toxic chemicals, they do impact our health.

2. Glyphosate functions as a chelator, meaning it holds or makes unavailable the vital nutrients of any living thing it touches. Reducing the nutrient content in our food supply is counter to good health and leads to mineral and vitamin deficiencies, which can cause illness and cancer. Farmers also report that herbicide tolerant GMO plants become "tougher" and, in the case of alfalfa, produce more fiber and less protein, which is the opposite of what farmers want for healthy livestock.

3. The manufacturer Monsanto first claimed that glyphosate-based herbicides only affect the shikimate pathway (a metabolic route used to produce essential folates and amino acids, which play a central role both as building blocks of proteins and with metabolism) in plants, which is not found in humans. What Monsanto failed to identify is that although the shikimate pathway is not found in our human cells, it *is* found in our gut bacteria, and thus is essential to maintain our good health. For every one human cell, ten bacteria are needed to maintain our bodily functions. Recently scientists have discovered that glyphosate herbicides *do* affect the shikimate pathway found in our gut bacteria, which is where our immune system lies.

What I am Calling DT or Desired Trait GMOs

The third kind of GMO is engineered to have a desired trait, like greener lettuce or a redder tomato. GMO proponents call them GMO 2.0—but I dislike the insinuation that they are somehow "better or improved" so I simply call them "Desired Trait" or DT GMOs. They do not include pesticide or herbicide tolerance, so they seem less harmful, but there are unknown risks to genetically modifying genes for any reason. These DT GMOs are listed by the hundreds in the United States Trademark and Patent Office. One can find them by searching for a type of seed and the word "promoter."

It is unknown if they are on the market currently because they are unlabeled. (GMOs are not required to be labeled in the USA.) We do know that the Simplot potatoes, the Arctic (non-browning) apple, the pink pineapple, Hawaiian papaya, and some varieties of zucchini and yellow crookneck squash are all examples of Desired Trait GMOs currently on the US market—but they are unlabeled. It should be noted that after twenty years of claiming GMOs are beneficial, there is not one GMO on the market that has provided any improved nutritional benefit to humans.

For example, RNAi GMO, causes an interference (hence the "i" in RNAi) with the genetic traits of a pest by inserting a microbe such as E. coli into the plant's RNA. It's like inserting chocolate chips into a sugar cookie recipe, along with a special code that allows the sugar cookie to "read" the chocolate chips. The insertion into the RNA could give it instructions to silence a mechanism, such as the browning function of an apple. Those promoters or silencers can wake genes up or silence certain functionalities in genes. The hope that the changes will not impact other functions of the life-form has yet to be proven true.

RNAi GMOs could be extremely dangerous because we, as parents or consumers, would have no idea if these promoters are waking up genes of rare diseases or if the silencers are silencing genes in our children or our own bodies. We would never have any way of knowing or proving if our child's rare disease or health issue was connected to GMOs. This unknown is unacceptable.

There are new genetic engineering technologies that are constantly being developed. The problem is that, as it currently stands, they will not be considered GMO and therefore not labeled—not even with a Quick Response (QR) code or symbol as the recently passed GMO labeling "law" requires. (Law is put in quotes because it is the opinion of the author that a law that does not require mandatory labeling, with wording on the package, is not a law. It is a farce.)

Nanotechnology

There are several types of nanotechnology. One concerning nano application in the food sector is nano-clay plastic polymers used as a coating to keep pesticide gasses from mixing with our food.

The Food Packaging Forum Foundation admits that "the migration potential of engineered nanomaterials (NMs) from food contact materials into food cannot be easily predicted. Even within one batch of nanoparticles, size may differ significantly, and the primary components of the nanoparticles may still remain in the mixture as impurities."

However, buying whole, organic, seasonal food from your farmer's market, Community Supported Agriculture (CSA), or co-op eliminates the need for or use of nanomaterials to protect from pesticide gassing and antimicrobials, and in addition you reduce plastic packaging in landfills.

Synthetic biology

Synthetic biology treats genes like computer code, remixing DNA sequences to create foods (and medicines, biofuels, and lots of other things) that do not occur in nature. Scientists are literally printing DNA and then placing that DNA in GMO yeast to create SynBio vanillin.

CRISPR technology

CRISPR/Cas9 genetic modification allows the permanent modification of genes within organisms. In other words, this type of genetic engineering can eliminate a genetic trait in an entire species forever—even in humans.

One might well ask: Who decides who gets to play God? Who decides what traits are or are not desirable? What are the ramifications of these decisions?

Dr. Vandana Shiva, world-renowned eco-activist, founder of Navdanya, and author of numerous books on ecology, recently discussed a study published in the journal Nature Methods May 30, 2017 issue showing that one gene edit resulted in over sixteen hundred mutations per mouse. Clearly, the ramifications are uncontrollable. She says, "GMOs are not an invention to be patented, they are a pollution of life." I agree.

Why Have GMOs and Toxins Been Allowed in Our Food?

> *"Someday we shall look back on this dark era of agriculture and shake our heads. How could we have ever believed that it was a good idea to grow our food with poisons?"*
> —DR. JANE GOODALL

Entire books have been written about the policy aspects of this issue (see lawyer Steven Drucker's book *Altered Genes Twisted Truth*, for one), but to sum up the primary ways the GMO chemical companies found a way to legally poison us, I give you this:

1. The GMO and chemical producers convinced the FDA to classify GMOs and pesticides as a "process" and not an "additive" to food. Had GMOs been considered an additive as well (which would make sense because you can test the foods and find them in the food after the process), they would have been required to be safety tested and labeled clearly on the package as required by law. The GMO and chemical manufacturers made very sure, early on, to make use of this loophole, tricking the entire American public into unknowingly eating GMOs and toxic chemicals and allowing these manufacturers to legally poison us.

2. How did they convince the FDA? The GMO and chemical companies made sure to have former loyal employees get jobs within the government regulatory agencies or in the White House. Michael Taylor, who formerly worked for Monsanto, was the deputy commissioner of the FDA during Obama's presidency. Having the fox guard the hen house is an understatement in our country. The fox is *in* the henhouse and is feasting away.

3. Why do so many people still not know about GMOs and toxins? Seventy percent of the commercials on mainstream TV networks are for pharmaceuticals. Big Pharma companies are actually the sister companies of Big Ag: agriculture companies, that is, GMO and chemical manufacturers. For example, DuPont, who makes GMOs and pesticides (that destroy beneficial bacteria in our gut), also owns Danisco, the largest US supplier of probiotics (which support healing our gut). These companies make us sick with their pesticides and then they "make us better" with their drugs. It's a perfect profit circle. Almost no major television network will risk losing their primary source of funding by running news about GMOs or pesticides that will upset their clients who are giving them millions in advertising dollars for the pharmaceutical commercials. Monsanto (currently in the process of merging with Bayer Pharmaceuticals formerly owned Pharmacia LLC a pharmaceutical company, now owned by Pfizer), Syngenta (sister company is Astra Zeneca biopharmaceuticals), and BASF all have the same story. I assert that their Big Pharma commercial dollars influence the mainstream media, so the public won't know the truth about

their Big Ag products, and they can continue to profit. Reporters and news outlet representatives have, in private, confirmed this theory and admitted to pulling or not publishing stories due to pressure from corporations such as Monsanto.

Next Steps

The more I learned, the more I felt betrayed by food manufacturers, grocers, the Food and Drug Administration (FDA), the United States Department of Agriculture (USDA), the Environmental Protection Agency (EPA), the Centers for Disease Control (CDC), and the White House. I felt duped, angry, frustrated, and frightened. I was truly afraid for the futures of my children. What if they ate the wrong food and I wasn't around to administer the EpiPen? What if they couldn't have children someday because of what I fed them? What if they got sick slowly and died in their twenties from cancer? I had heard of more and more young people in their twenties getting colitis, Crohn's disease, and stomach cancer, more and more wives and mothers dying in their thirties from breast cancer, and more and more husbands and fathers in their forties dying suddenly . . . leaving families behind with young children who were devastated.

I began to have an overwhelming awareness that the genetic engineering of food was the underlying cause for the majority of these rising health issues. What Jeffrey Smith was saying in his movie seemed so surreal, though, so incredibly scary that our government would allow this to happen that I didn't talk about it with others at first. There is a fine line between discovering information, being savvy, and appearing to be totally paranoid. I didn't want people to think I was a conspiracy theorist and write me off as a nutter. I didn't want to alienate myself from my friends. So, I didn't tell them at first. I sat in my fear for three days. The very thing I wanted to avoid was the thing I ended up being—alone.

After three days, I emailed my family and best friend and asked them to please watch the TEDx Talk and *Genetic Roulette*. I posted Robyn's video on Facebook and, after a few days, I began to share information about GMOs with my circle of close friends. They were shocked. Many didn't know what to say. Some were angry. None of us knew what to do or where to go to for help. We were stopped from taking action by our fear of the unknown. What do we do now?

There is a saying that goes, "A worried mom does better research than the FBI." Because my children had health issues that I suspected were connected to the changes in the food supply, once again, I began to research.

I pored through technical information from many global experts and soon realized one did not need to be a rocket scientist to understand what was going on. Moms like Holly nicely summed up GMOs:

> Ideally, it would be better to not just label GM foods but also to ban them as other countries have done.
>
> - GM food has new proteins that people haven't encountered before and that some people can't digest.
>
> - GM food contains built-in pesticides, which we eat.
>
> - GM crops are designed to tolerate greater amounts of herbicide, and that herbicide pollutes our soil and water.
>
> - GM crops cut down on biodiversity.
>
> - GM crops contaminate non-GM crops.
>
> - Monsanto has patents on seeds. Come on!

There were already hundreds, if not over a thousand, of studies by the fall of 2013—the peak of the GMO labeling campaign—that demonstrated the harm that could be done by GMOs. I learned that when goats were fed GMOs, the mother goat produced less milk and thus the kid's health was impacted. The third generation of rats was sterile when the mother ate GMOs. Hamsters were smaller and failed to thrive when they ate GMOs. I didn't need any more scientific studies to convince me that GMOs were not in a mother's, or a child's, best interest.

I shared this information with my husband and kids and we agreed to avoid GMOs. I saw significant health changes in my eldest son. I went to a showing of *Genetic Roulette* (even though I had already seen it), met some great people, and signed up to be a volunteer for Prop 37, the California Labeling Initiative instigated by grandmother and midwife Pamm Larry.

Getting involved in the initiative was scary at first, but also inspiring. I no longer felt alone, and the dedication of the people supporting the initiative compelled me to learn and do more. I will never forget the patience, passion, and energy of volunteer coordinators Kerne, Paula, and John, who motivated me to take the cause on as my own. When we lost the ballot initiative, my commitment was not deterred, and I pledged to keep going. My first step into leadership, however, was within my own family.

CHAPTER THREE

LEARNING THE TRUTH ABOUT GLYPHOSATE

"From now on I'll connect the dots my own way."
—BILL WATTERSON

AFTER MOMS ACROSS America's first big event, joining into Fourth of July parades in 2013 (which I will discuss later), I was on the East Coast visiting my family. I decided to call on Anthony Samsel, an independent scientist in New Hampshire who was working with MIT scientist Dr. Stephanie Seneff. I knew even then that their work was controversial, and that I might be criticized for sharing it (I was). Their type of science, which is more theoretical, connects the dots between many existing studies, rather than, for instance, doing one study with two thousand rats that takes three years. This type of work is important in raising questions whose answers could help moms like me to avoid chemicals that could cause our children harm right now—years before harm from the chemicals are proven by other scientists in a lab with animal testing.

I wanted to interview Dr. Samsel about glyphosate, the declared active chemical ingredient in Roundup, which 80 percent of GMOs were engineered to withstand. I knew that GMOs themselves were a huge problem, but I had a growing suspicion that glyphosate herbicides were an even bigger problem than was being recognized. I had a feeling that GMOs and the toxic chemicals used in conjunction with them, or pesticides alone used on non-organic crops, were *equally* harmful or—possibly—that the chemicals were even more harmful.

Samsel, one of the few experts in the field of glyphosate research at the time, began to walk me through the world of glyphosate-based herbicides.

First, he explained how detrimental glyphosate is to the human body and life on the planet. He did not mince words.

"There should be zero glyphosate in our food and water. It is an insidiously harmful chemical and should be completely banned," he told me.

Below, based on discussions that I had with Samsel and Dr. Stephanie Seneff of MIT, who has co-authored with Samsel and has also independently written many papers on glyphosate, is a description of how glyphosate functions and why they feel glyphosate herbicides are connected to dozens of modern diseases.

- Glyphosate is scientifically accepted to function as a chelator, which draws out the vital nutrients of any living thing it touches. This leads to a deficiency of rare minerals like manganese, cobalt, molybdenum, copper, iron, sulfur, and selenium. Without the necessary minerals, we cannot fight cancer or manage the very important nutrients throughout the body. The minerals pile up in the wrong places, causing both toxicity and deficiency at the same time.

- Glyphosate is an antimicrobial agent (a patented antibiotic) and it preferentially kills the good bacteria, which causes an overgrowth of pathogens in the gut. This leads to leaky gut syndrome and inflammatory issues. Seventy percent of the immune system lies in the gut biome. Destroying the gut bacteria impairs the body's ability to create tryptophan/serotonin, and melatonin, which regulate insulin/diabetes and protect from sleeplessness, depression, bipolar disorder, and violent behavior. As an antibiotic, glyphosate has also been shown to increase antibiotic resistance, leading to superbugs such as E. coli and salmonella, which can be deadly.

- Glyphosate disrupts cytochrome P450 enzymes' function in the liver, which is important for many things, two of which are activating vitamin D and detoxifying multiple toxic chemicals and drugs. Acetaminophen (Tylenol), for example, becomes toxic when these enzymes aren't working. Not a good combination for a baby to have glyphosate in breast milk and then be given Tylenol for teething pain or a fever.

- Glyphosate interferes with the shikimate pathway, which is used by both microbes and plants to produce essential aromatic amino acids. Our own cells don't have this pathway, so they depend on food sources and synthesis by gut microbes to supply these nutrients. They are precursors to many biologically important molecules such as the neurotransmitters serotonin, melatonin, dopamine, norepinephrine, melanin, vitamin E, vitamin K, and more.

  I also learned from Don Huber, Michael Antoniou, Gilles-Éric Séralini and the CRIIGEN team, Howard Vlieger, and many other experts about the potential harm of glyphosate herbicides. Even though we had been told glyphosate was as safe as table salt, studies were revealing otherwise.

- Dr. Matt Buckley, inspired by Samsel and Seneff's work, described to me how glyphosate targets beneficial gut bacteria and promotes the proliferation of pathogenic bacteria such as E. coli and salmonella. This can lead to increased urinary tract infections and gut dysbiosis. Pathogenic gut bacteria prompt the vagus nerve in the gut to signal the microglial cells in the brain to go on "attack." The attack means that the microglial cells can create glutamate, an excitotoxin, which excites the brain neurons and eventually causes brain neuron death. This could lead to autism symptoms such as ticks, stammers, repetitive behavior, as well as brain fog, dementia, and Alzheimer's.

- UK scientist Michael Antoniou, Ph.D., taught me that at low levels, glyphosate herbicides are proven to be endocrine disruptors, which may impact, deform, or halt the development of a fetus leading to miscarriage, and also may cause birth defects, infertility, and sterility at minute levels. Dose does not make the poison in the case of endocrine disruptors. Tiny amounts can deform—or even be fatal to—a fetus.

- In a test commissioned by Moms Across America, glyphosate was found in all five childhood vaccines tested at an accredited lab, and dozens of others by a different, independent lab and the results were confirmed. Seneff argues that glyphosate could be working synergistically with the aluminum, mercury, and glutamate in vaccines to cause much greater harm than would be the case if there was no glyphosate present in the blood when the vaccine was administered. Glyphosate herbicide is a cell disintegrator that breaks down the blood-brain barrier and allows toxins into the brain. The timing of the introduction of glyphosate into the food supply correlates with the rise of autism as closely as 99 percent. The FDA has not responded to Moms Across America's requests to test and confirm the presence of glyphosate in vaccines.

- Gilles-Éric Séralini's team in France discovered that the co-formulants, or other ingredients in Roundup besides glyphosate, are up to one thousand times more toxic than glyphosate alone. The EPA only requires the one declared active chemical ingredient to be tested, however—not the final formulation.

- New studies find that glyphosate also feeds antibiotic-resistant bacteria, which can lead to methicillin-resistant Staphylococcus aureus (MRSA) and other serious contagious diseases that are on the rise.

- A report was released in January 2017, by scientists Antoniou, Mesange et al. that Roundup causes nonalcoholic fatty liver disease (NAFLD) at levels far lower than what is allowed in our food. According to the American Liver Foundation, one out of ten Americans currently has NAFLD.

- The Monsanto Papers, released by Baum, Hedlund, Aristei & Goldman in the fall of 2017, revealed an admission by Monsanto that glyphosate not only contains but also forms nitrosamines in the body, which are compounds that generally cause cancer.

- Glyphosate herbicides and GMOs have been shown to be tumorigenic, meaning causing tumors, by French scientist Séralini and his team in a two-year (lifetime of the rats) study. This paper was retracted by the journal that originally published it after a former Monsanto employee joined the staff. The critics deemed the study invalid because Séralini used "rats prone to cancer," failing to disclose that Séralini's team chose those particular rats because Monsanto had used them in their three-month study. It was later discovered by independent scientists that all the lab rat chow tested was contaminated with glyphosate, invalidating all previous studies with control groups that were supposed to be eating food without glyphosate. Therefore, all previous studies that claimed there was no significant difference in an increase of tumors or health issues with animals would need to be redone with control groups eating glyphosate-free food in order for the results to be considered valid. This has not happened, and the EPA continues to allow glyphosate herbicides to be used without valid studies proving their safety.

From his farm in New Hampshire, Samsel also told me that it was not just GMOs that were being sprayed with glyphosate, but that hundreds of non-GMO crops had high residue levels because the farmers were being encouraged to spray glyphosate as a desiccant (drying agent) before harvest. Glyphosate was also sprayed as a burn down before planting, and crops such as carrots, potatoes, and berries then uptake the chemical through their roots. He showed me the list on the EPA website of the 160 food crops and their allowable levels of glyphosate. I felt like I had been punched in the gut.

I knew that a study by Monika Kruger et al. showed that glyphosate had destroyed gut bacteria (which weakens the immune system) in chickens at 0.1 ppm (part per million) and a study by Thongprakaisang et al. stimulated the growth of breast cancer cells in vitro (human cells) at only one part per trillion (ppt). One ppt is equivalent to one drop in the water of twenty-two Olympic-size swimming pools combined. Yet the EPA allows levels in the hundreds of parts per million—thousands of times higher—in our food and water. In addition, it has been shown that glyphosate both bioaccumulates and is an endocrine disruptor, which means that at minuscule amounts it can cause harm—so, therefore, any amount is harmful.

GMO chemical farming proponents claim that GMOs have decreased the amount of pesticides used, but if you consider that the term pesticide is widely considered to include herbicides, which are just as toxic, then this statement is false. GMO chemical farming has, in fact, dramatically increased the use of pesticides. The EPA reported in 2015 that between 2004 and 2013, on average every year 1.1 million pounds of glyphosate was sprayed on sunflower seeds, 1.3 million on sugar beets, 3.2 million on oranges, 2.1 on almonds, 8.6 million on wheat, 18.5 million on cotton/cottonseed (used in oil), 63.5 million on corn crops, and 101 million pounds of glyphosate was used on soybeans. In 2014, a recorded three hundred million pounds of glyphosate herbicides were used in the USA. Fifty years ago? Zero. A study released in October of 2017 showed that elderly adults in Southern California were exposed to 500 percent more glyphosate over a thirteen-year period and excreted in urine over one thousand times more glyphosate than their initial screening.

Below is just a sample of some food crops and what the EPA says are their allowable glyphosate residues:

Animal Feed, Grains	400 ppm
Berries	0.2 ppm
Carrots and Potatoes	5 ppm
Canola and Soy	20 ppm
Corn	13 ppm
Grass, Forage, Fodder	200 ppm
Grains, Wheat, Buckwheat, Sorghum	30 ppm
Legumes, Quinoa	5 ppm
Nuts, Tree	1 ppm
Sweet Potatoes	5 ppm
Wheat	30 ppm
Sugar	25 ppm
Sunflower and Safflower Oil	85 ppm
Tea	7 ppm

I left the meeting with Samsel in despair. I knew that we had to raise awareness, not just about GMOs to transform the food supply, but also about glyphosate and the entire system of chemical farming. Suddenly, my mission was bigger—and seemed more daunting than ever.

Learning from All Sides

After I learned more about glyphosate, others involved in the cause began to insist that we were in a fight over the food supply, and one activist suggested I read the book *The Art of War* by Sun Tzu. I was hesitant to think in these terms, but I felt it best to prepare myself by whatever means necessary for the huge task before me. In Tzu's book I learned about strategy, the benefit of silence, and approaches I never would have considered before. One strategy is to study your opponent, get in their shoes, and think like they think. So, I began to watch the videos and read information put out by the pro-GMO proponents.

In a pro-GMO panel discussion at the Heritage Foundation, a woman on the panel declared that the food industry's biggest problem was the growing number of "mom bloggers" who claimed that their children get better when they avoid GMOs. She argued that they were fraudulently misleading the American public. She asserted that they had no scientific evidence. Bells went off. I knew I needed to gather scientific evidence.

We had to test for glyphosate in our children. We had to show the GMO companies that their products were in our children and our bodies and to be able to make a connection between that and their health issues. I asked my doctor and six different labs—none could test for glyphosate. Not one doctor even knew what it was. One lab said there were no tests for glyphosate because it was considered safe. I told them that asbestos and lead were considered safe at one time, too . . . we needed to test anyway. But they did not have the ability to do so. I appealed to the only person that I thought might know someone who could actually do something. A farmer.

Glyphosate in My Son

A few months after learning about glyphosate, my eight-year-old son Bodee, previously a happy go-getter, began exhibiting erratic behavior. He was screaming, had learning issues, rashes, very smelly urine, was bedwetting, and was even aggressive toward my husband and me. His teacher called and expressed serious concern, saying that he was not doing his work and was giving up. His grades dropped from As to Ds and Fs. I asked him why and he said, "It's just too hard. I hate it." This was a boy who had previously enjoyed being at the top of his class. Suddenly, he was turning in quizzes with ten questions, after answering only one question and writing -9 at the top, willingly failing.

My husband hoped it was just a phase . . . but I saw a look in my son's eyes, behind the rage, even while he was trying to hit me, that said, "*Help me.* I do not want to be this way." I knew there was something else going on.

I took Bodee to our doctor, who happened to be a doctor who specializes in treating autism. I liked the spaced-out vaccine schedule that he supported, although at the time Bodee had not had a vaccine in three years. The doctor said he would test my son for fungus and bacteria in his urine. When I asked him why fungus, he said, "Because sometimes fungus and an overgrowth of pathogenic bacteria in the gut can cause inflammation in the brain and affect behavior." Bells went off. That's what glyphosate does! It kills the beneficial gut bacteria and promotes the pathogenic gut bacteria, thereby causing inflammation in the brain! My doctor and I had a forty-five-minute discussion. He said I should speak at the Medical Academy of Pediatric Special Needs (MAPS) conference in front of nationally recognized doctors. I would not be able to, as I am not an MD, but his willingness to learn from me shows the need for a shift in the perspective of caring for our children. Doctors need to listen to mothers. We mothers should no longer just blindly trust our Western medical doctors. They don't know everything. In fact, in many cases, they are taught almost nothing in medical school about the *causes* of the issues currently affecting our children and the ways to resolve them. Those who want to get to the source and try solutions other than pharmaceutical drugs and synthetic chemicals need to log their child's symptoms and seek out integrative medicine and alternative therapies. Dedicated parents who research the possible causes of health problems, are willing to try new things, and are open to natural remedies and diet can provide a crucial part of the solution.

My son's urine tested extremely high for fungus and pathogenic gut bacteria—even the deadly clostridium difficile (C. diff), which can lead to colitis. I was extremely alarmed. His doctor said he had autism symptoms because of the gut dysbiosis, holes in his small intestine, and over twenty different food intolerances. I was utterly distraught. We had been feeding him non-GMO food for almost two years . . . why was this happening? Were Bodee's learning issues somehow connected to glyphosate?

At the same time that we learned of Bodee's health issues, pestering a farmer friend to find a lab that would test for glyphosate paid off. He emailed me the name of a lab. Moms Across America would be able to start glyphosate testing! For the first time in this country, people would be able to test their urine and tap water for glyphosate. It was very exciting—and scary at the same time. I was terrified to find out how much glyphosate was in my sons, but also determined to get to the truth and then take action to resolve their health issues. I sent and paid for all three of my sons' and my own urine to be tested (my husband didn't feel the need) and encouraged others to do the same.

Within a few hours, in December of 2013, the infographic that Moms Across America shared to encourage glyphosate testing of urine and tap water reached thirty-three thousand people.

Forty people sent in their samples, paid for their own testing, and agreed to share their results with us anonymously so we could inform the public of the results. The majority of the tap water samples came back positive—at low levels, but still of concern. I was infuriated but not surprised to learn that my tap water, in Orange County, California had .087 ppb of glyphosate in it. I later learned that the various state water resource departments and United States Geological Surveys show that Roundup is being sprayed around water reservoirs and has been detected in the majority of our water supplies across the nation, including farm irrigation. Roundup has been linked to an increased growth of toxic algae in reservoirs, which in turn has caused the Department of Water Resources to commission the aerial spraying of copper sulfate into the reservoirs to eliminate the algae. Copper is a known spermicide. Glyphosate herbicide has been shown to increase the harmful impact of toxins and metals. Obviously, increasing the level of spermicidal copper in our water is of huge concern. New studies show that the rates of sperm quality in men in the United States has dropped *59 percent over the past forty years*, since glyphosate herbicides were first introduced into our agriculture system.

I immediately installed a reverse osmosis system under my kitchen sink and retested our water. This time the results came back not detectable for glyphosate above .05 ppb, which put me somewhat at ease.

The urine test results from the forty samples the public sent in during our campaign were alarming. A college student with cancer tested as high as 19 ppb.

My eldest son's and my youngest son's and my urine tested negative, but my middle son's levels came back 8.75 ppb, which was eight times higher than had been found in anyone tested in Europe. Glyphosate weed killer was in *my son's* body! I was furious! I remember running down the stairs filled with rage, calling my husband and crying to him over the phone. I couldn't tell anyone, post it online, or speak about it until all our data was in and I could write up a report that would be seen as legitimate. I was frustrated, angry, and desperate for a way to help my son. This had to be connected to his high levels of fungus and bacteria. This had to be connected to his behavior issues and radical health decline.

Bodee was the only one of my three boys who had not tested positive for a gluten intolerance, and therefore he was the only one who ate conventional wheat now and then. When we went to a restaurant or to a friend's home, which was about once or twice a week, we let him eat a burger with a bun, pizza, or a burrito with a wheat-flour wrap. I realized that I was allowing him to eat wheat that was being heavily sprayed with glyphosate as a drying agent. Residues of glyphosate were expected to be high, since the EPA allows up to 30 ppm on wheat and grains. Scientists were beginning to attribute leaky gut to glyphosate herbicides destroying the gut bacteria, and even though I did not have peer-reviewed, scientific proof, I had a very strong suspicion about wheat that I could not ignore.

I felt horrible. All this time, I thought that going GMO-free was good enough (wheat is not GMO), and that not eating organic *all* the time would be okay. But no, I said to myself. *This is it.* I will not be a part of giving even a small amount of poison to my family. The expression "everything in moderation" simply does not work with poison. Even the 80/20 rule does not work if the 20 percent is slowly destroying my child's health.

So, we went 100 percent organic—even our meat—and followed the doctor's instructions to eliminate the fungus and bacteria in Bodee's gut with a $650 a month antifungal medication and antibiotic. My son also agreed not to eat any sugar between Thanksgiving and New Year's. He accomplished this astonishing feat to prevent feeding the bad bacteria. We gave him sauerkraut, (loaded with good bacteria), colloidal silver, and lots of green smoothies. Six weeks later, we retested him. His glyphosate levels were no longer detectable, and his autism symptoms were gone. They have never come back.

No one can put a price tag on the cost of the hardship a family goes through with a child of autism. TV shows and movies that portray high functioning teens with autism do not show the reality of thousands of families who are dealing with much more difficult—even violent—situations. If you don't personally know parents of a severely autistic child, you don't know that they often live in fear of being beaten up by their own child, of having their child arrested for violent behavior in public, or of their child inflicting harm on his or herself hundreds of times a day. Even mildly autistic children with learning and behavioral issues can cause a great strain on marriages, as parents often blame themselves or each other—resulting in divorce, addictions, or depression. Siblings of children with autism are also greatly impacted. Their needs often go ignored and their view of the world sours when they see their sibling being bullied for his or her differences. The struggle of the family dealing with autism is indescribable.

Also, the financial burden of autism is often crippling. Mothers of children with autism have informed me that they spend $65,000–$100,000 a year on therapies and medication for their child's care. They often leave their careers to stay home and care for their child, cutting the household income—often by half. When people tell me eating organic food is too expensive, I adamantly deny it.

In addition to our relief at my son's autism symptoms disappearing, I estimate that by going organic and restoring his gut biome, that we have saved at least $260,000 in four years. Organic food is far cheaper than doctor's bills. It's not too expensive. It's more nutritious, has far fewer toxins, and is better for the environment. In fact, as a nation, I would go so far to say that we cannot afford to *not* eat organic.

Testing for Glyphosate

After seeing such an improvement in my son's health, I immediately wanted to know what else in our lives that glyphosate was contaminating. The lab could not test for food yet, so I asked about beverages and bodily fluids. In addition to water, I really wanted to know if glyphosate was in breast milk and semen but didn't know how to get samples and thought I couldn't get enough of them. When Sustainable Pulse (an international GMO news website) director Henry Rowlands Skyped me and asked if his organization could fund the testing of 100 samples of breast milk for glyphosate, I was thrilled. I had to find a way. The implications of the results could be huge. In fact, Rowlands pointed out that dichlorodiphenyltrichloroethane (DDT) and polychlorinated biphenyl (PCB's), both made by Monsanto, were found in women's breast milk and within five years of these results they were banned. I knew that *this could be it*. I had to get it done. I contacted every breast milk bank I could find for a month. No one would agree to participate. I then decided I had to be able to find at least ten mom supporters who would help.

I sat down and started calling moms across the country. Finally, three weeks later, ten moms had sent in their samples by FedEx directly to the lab, paying for the shipping themselves and agreeing to let me publish the results anonymously. It was a courageous thing for them to donate their breast milk. What do you do if it is positive? How horrible is it to think you are feeding your child weed killer? It's unthinkable. I truly honor those brave women who sent their breast milk samples to be tested. (We hope to get funding and donors to test semen soon as well.)

After the breast milk samples reached the lab, the staff let us know that the glyphosate levels would have to be above 75 ppb to be detectable, as the methodology was new, and it was the best they could do. This was far higher than the .05 ppb for water. I was very disappointed by this high level of detectability. I was sure that we would not find any glyphosate above this level, and although that would be a good result, the test results would not help our cause to raise awareness. Nor would it give us a true understanding of whether glyphosate was actually present or not.

A few weeks later the results came back. I was shocked. Three of the ten samples were positive for glyphosate, even though nine out of ten of the women were supporters of Moms Across America and were actively avoiding GMOs and glyphosate in their food. The positive levels were 76 ppb, 99 ppb, and 166 ppb. Incredible. The two moms who had 76 ppb and 99 ppb admitted to eating out (conventional food) a few times a week. The mother that had 166 ppb, the highest level, was a friend of an MAA supporter, and did not know about GMOs or glyphosate and therefore ate the standard American diet. The 166 ppb was three thousand times higher than has been shown to cause sex hormone changes and causes harm to rats in Séralini's study. I was, again, outraged. Henry Rowlands wrote up the report and, after having a few scientists comment on the results, we published the report on the Moms Across America website and Sustainable Pulse. I sent a letter to the EPA with the results and asked them to recall Roundup, as the manufacturer had claimed that glyphosate would not enter breast milk, but pass harmlessly through the body and be expelled in urine. Clearly, the product wasn't doing what the manufacturer said it would do, and therefore it needed to be recalled.

After a month of no response from the EPA, we were furious. In one group phone call, several moms decided to start a five-day call campaign to the federal and regional EPA offices. I found the telephone numbers, the Moms

Across America's graphic designer Anne Temple made a Facebook event with a map of the EPA office locations and the phone numbers, a few memes, and we started spreading the campaign on social media. We called the EPA every day—both the local and federal offices. By the third day, an EPA staffer told a supporter that he had to get these women to stop calling them—that over ten thousand women had called in three days. By the fifth day, the EPA pesticide review branch manager was not exactly calm when we spoke. He said he needed us to stop calling so that they could do their jobs.

I told him, "Your job is to recall Roundup, and we won't stop."

He suggested that a "meeting with principals" would be more effective, so we arranged to meet a week and a half later in Washington, DC, when I would happen to be on the East Coast for a demonstration and conference. Coincidentally, we later found out that the day of our meeting with the EPA, May 27, was the birthday of Rachel Carson, author of *Silent Spring*. She predicted all the troubles that we are now experiencing with toxins, and the government created the EPA in response. How serendipitous to meet with them on her birthday.

According to the EPA's website: "The EPA regulates the production and distribution of commercial and industrial chemicals to ensure that chemicals made available for sale and use in the United States *do not harm human health or the environment.*"

The problem is, they are not doing their job.

Over eighty thousand chemicals have been approved by the EPA since the 1940s, and only nine have been banned. A paper published in 2016 showed that in 2010, the United States had $42 billion in costs from organophosphate pesticide endocrine disruptors (Roundup's classification). None of the chemical products approved for use have been approved in their final formulation state—only one ingredient has been safety tested. This major flaw in the system makes the EPA completely ineffective. They have to be held accountable.

The meeting with the EPA was necessary but astounding to me. How was it that *I* was going to meet with the EPA? I knew very well why—but it still seemed surreal. When word got out, the food movement community rallied in an extraordinary way. Scientists, health-care providers, and lawyers from major nonprofits joined me. A grandmother and former marine along with several moms also showed up, spoke up, and demanded action. There were eleven of us and nine EPA staffers and people from across the country listening to the meeting live. The EPA staffers were glued to their seats and the meeting went two hours instead of one, with not one person attempting to leave. The experiences the other moms shared of their children's health declining when they ate food with glyphosate residue, and of their health improving when they did not, were strong and clear. I did not preselect the women for their experiences—they just cared, showed up, and spoke up. I saw denial and anger in some of the EPA staffers' faces, but I also saw empathy, curiosity, and concern for others. I believe we made a difference—even though they still have not released the tests for glyphosate in breast milk as they said they would. In other countries, the breast milk testing had a greater impact. Without the courage of the ten women who sent in their breast milk samples, I dare say I do not think that entire countries would currently be banning glyphosate.

Subsequently, Monsanto funded testing for glyphosate in breast milk as well and . . . surprise, surprise, did not find any. The co-authors of the paper, Shelly and Mark McGuire, professed to have no connection to Monsanto whatsoever. It was later revealed, however, by Valerie Brown and the late Elizabeth Grossman, reporters for *In These Times,* that both Shelly and Mark had strong ties to Monsanto and were, in fact, each "gifted" $10,000 by the chemical company. Interestingly enough, Shelly and Mark McGuire did not follow the standard scientific practice of duplicating the testing exactly. They used a different methodology—and some scientists are now questioning that methodology and its ability to detect the glyphosate inside protein cells (where it could hide). Even the FDA halted testing for glyphosate in 2016 due to concerns over the reliability of this testing methodology. Which calls to the forefront an even bigger question: Why, if glyphosate is so difficult to detect, and it cannot be accurately regulated, is the FDA permitting it to be sprayed on our food crops in the first place? Why wasn't methodology developed more than forty years ago, before it was allowed to be used in our food supply? I assert that if a chemical cannot be accurately detected and regulated, it must be pulled from the market.

In 2014, glyphosate was also found to enter the human bloodstream. A study by Kwiatkowska et al. found that glyphosate and other ingredients in Roundup lead to "slightly significant" negative effects on red blood cells. In other words, our blood is simply not Roundup ready and glyphosate does not pass "harmlessly through the body and is excreted in urine" as Monsanto has claimed.

Later in 2016, concerned about harm to our most vulnerable babies and children, we raised enough funds to test twenty baby formulas and twenty PediaSure feeding tube liquid samples. Although our baby formula samples did not detect positive above 75 ppb (which does not mean that it was not present at lower levels), Samsel did find positive levels up to 170 ppb in soy Enfamil baby formula—even higher than in breast milk.

The detectable level of glyphosate was 75 ppb. Six of the PediaSure Enteral feeding tube liquid samples tested positive over 75 ppb. Séralini has shown that only 50 ppt (parts per trillion) of glyphosate was shown to cause liver, kidney, and sex hormone changes in rats. PediaSure Enteral Formula, made by Abbott, is the exact brand used in the pediatric rehabilitation hospital where a Moms Across America supporter worked, and it was fed to patients needing tube feeding in critical care.

I found it appalling that our health-care providers have been led to believe this feeding tube liquid is safe. Our children and loved ones who are depending on our health-care institutions to support their immune systems and recoveries are instead being fed a liquid that scientists and informed caregivers now believe is doing the exact opposite. The PediaSure Enteral Formula tested is loaded with genetically modified corn syrup, soy, and sugar—which have all been shown to cause inflammation.

Several scientists and notable food advocates commented on the finding of glyphosate in the feeding tube liquid and the ubiquitous contamination of glyphosate.

> *As a mother, I am very disturbed by these results. Working as a pediatric physical therapist, I meet children with feeding issues who depend on tube feedings for their entire lives. Children who experience trauma and are recovering from car accidents, shootings, surgeries, cancers, and other illnesses may require these tube feedings for days, weeks, or years. I have long questioned the nutritionally poor and inflammatory ingredients in these feedings but am devastated to find out that they are contaminated with poison. Our most vulnerable children, and our children healing from overwhelming trauma, deserve better.* —SARAH CUSACK, MPT, CHHC

> *Glyphosate in PediaSure is frightening. As a cardiologist concerned about herbicides, I now know that Roundup affects heart tissue and*

facilitates serious heart rhythm problems. To think we are exposing infants to this same toxin cannot be tolerated. —Joel Kahn, MD

I find it astonishing that babies and children with cancer are being provided with nutrients through a feeding tube that is contaminated with glyphosate. It ought to be obvious to medical professionals that it is essential to assure that as few toxic chemicals as possible are present in enteral nutrition provided to seriously ill children. This is a direct delivery system for glyphosate to the blood and to the tissues. It should be undeniable that certified organic sources are the only viable option in such a situation.

—Stephanie Seneff, MIT scientist and coauthor of the "Glyphosate Papers"

The release of the glyphosate findings in our children's urine, tap water, and especially breast milk caused a global stir. Later people from Switzerland, China, and Hawai'i told me that those findings brought a new life to their movement. Exposing the truth is powerful. I am very grateful to the women who made those tests possible, to Sustainable Pulse for the funding, to the farmer who asked the lab to do the testing, and to the owner of the lab Microbe Inotech.

The test results from the PediaSure feeding tube liquid, however, got almost no media. It was too awful, I think, to imagine that children with cancer were being fed weed killer. It infuriated me that the media would pick up stories of movie stars having affairs, but they would not publish a story to expose the poisoning of our most vulnerable children. All I could do was keep going.

In March 2015, our community got a huge surprise when the World Health Organization (WHO), a branch of the United Nations, and the International Agency for Research on Cancer (IARC), deemed glyphosate to be a Class 2 probable carcinogen. Not long afterward, Samsel announced that he had acquired over ten thousand pages of Monsanto studies and documents from the EPA with the help of his senator. In those documents, there is evidence that Monsanto had known that glyphosate was carcinogenic and harmful to life since the early 1980s. Since then, studies showing a 50 percent increase of non-Hodgkin lymphoma due to exposure to Roundup have surfaced. Lawsuits have followed. The pro-GMO and chemical company proponents have refused to acknowledge harm, however, and have vilified anyone who provided the truth to the public.

Michael K. Hansen, Ph.D. senior staff scientist at the policy and advocacy division of *Consumer Reports*, kindly supported me in preparation for the California EPA Office of Environmental Health Hazard Assessment (OEHHA) meeting on July 7, 2017, on the "no significant risk level" of glyphosate using the EPA's levels. We worked out the daily intake of glyphosate herbicide by a typical American child based on the detected levels found by many different consumer advocate groups, and the residue amounts allowed by the EPA. These levels were alarming. An average twenty-two-pound toddler is, typically, according to test results, consuming 2.2 times more glyphosate and could, according to the EPA, consume nearly six times more than the California EPA was proposing (1,100 micrograms per day, per food item) as being a safe level. These levels are thousands of times higher than has been shown to cause harm such as liver disease. The US federal levels are even worse. The US federal acceptable daily intake (ADI) is seventeen times higher than the European ADI of 0.3 mg/kg. At 1.75 mg/kg, the EPA ADI only takes into consideration a 175-pound adult, not a baby, so these levels are clearly not safe. Americans deserve better.

In 2015, the nonprofit organization GMO Free USA tested foods for glyphosate, and exposed high levels in America's most popular breakfast cereals. In 2016, the Alliance for Natural Health tested breakfast foods—and eggs, bagels, milk, and yogurt were all found to be positive. Even the FDA tested honey and oatmeal, which were positive for glyphosate above the allowable levels. According to a study by the Socio-Environmental Interaction Space (EMISA) of the University of La Plata, Argentina, cotton swabs, wipes, tampons, and sanitary pads were also found to contain glyphosate and aminomethylphosphonic acid (AMPA), the residual breakdown of glyphosate—which can be even more toxic.

In March 2016, a Moms Across America supporter gave me glyphosate test results for twelve California wines, which were all positive. I wrote up the report, and that news did make the media. I filmed a segment for ABC7 in San Francisco. The first piece aired, and it was exciting to learn that they would be airing a second segment with more information on ABC's *World News Tonight* on that Saturday. Then I learned that Monsanto had sent a memo to the station, and the second segment was cancelled. Our moms were very upset and began calling and emailing the station. I sent a letter directly to Monsanto. Something worked. The second segment was aired later in the week, and millions more learned about glyphosate in wine.

Sustainable Pulse and Food Democracy Now tested a large batch of snacks, crackers, and chips in the fall of 2016, and the majority were found to be positive at levels hundreds of times higher than has been shown to destroy gut bacteria.

The findings in our food supply made news with RT.com (Russia Today), one of the only news outlets that has been covering the truth about our food. It is no secret that the Russian President, Vladimir Putin, hates GMOs. He has banned GMOs from his country and disallowed GMO imports. It is possible that he may have another political agenda besides protecting his people—but regardless, we appreciated the news coverage.

Then, astonishingly, the Canadian Food Inspection Agency (CFIA) tested thousands of food samples for glyphosate primarily from North America but also from several other countries around the world. The credit must go to the UNSTOPPABLE efforts of Tony Mitra, a tenacious Canadian activist who barraged his government with emails and requests for testing. Once they had done the testing, Tony assembled the 7,800 test results in his book *Poison Foods of North America*. These shocking results showed that anywhere from 50 to 100 percent of certain types of food were positive for glyphosate in the United States—specifically lentils, millet, wheat/soy/bean flours, chickpeas, oats, and pizza products. Even some organic samples tested positive. Some, like organic garbanzo beans and organic red lentils from North America, had glyphosate levels almost as high as their conventional counterparts, pointing to fraudulent organic labeling.

Reports of imported conventional foods from Turkey suddenly being labeled "organic" at the ports were exposed in 2017. Of course, this brings all organic foods into question. I have found however, from reviewing thousands of glyphosate tests, that most food that is labeled organic is not contaminated—and that if it is, the levels are on average twenty-six times lower than conventional. Organic is still is the best we have. The garbanzo beans and lentils in the CFIA testing are a mysterious anomaly. Until further testing is done, and organic standards are enforced, I would suggest getting your garbanzo beans or hummus and red lentils from a source other than North America. I would suggest that those who want to take a step further get involved with the National Organic Standards Board (NOSB) meetings and speak up for better enforcement from our USDA.

Canadian glyphosate residue levels were the highest, which makes sense when you consider that the weather is wetter than in the US, and farmers use more glyphosate as a drying agent in wetter regions. Not so coincidentally, perhaps, Canada has the highest rates of irritable bowel syndrome (IBS) in the world.

In May 2017, Séralini's team was supposed to publish a study revealing that arsenic and heavy metals were detected in all the glyphosate-based herbicides tested. However, the study was delayed by the journal that was going to publish it as well as the regulators, and Séralini stated that he was sure it was to prevent the European decision makers from learning this information and revoking the license of glyphosate in the fall of 2017. The EU renewed the license for another five years. In January 2018, the study finally came out, and citizens and policymakers alike were shocked to learn that levels of arsenic in glyphosate herbicides were five to 100 times higher than what is allowed in the water supply. This poison and endocrine disrupting heavy metals were being sprayed on our food crops or in our gardens.

Not only is the discovery of arsenic and heavy metals in Roundup at dangerously toxic levels and glyphosate-based herbicides extremely disturbing, because these ingredients were not declared, *the manufacturers could be liable for fraud.* Professor Gilles-Éric Séralini comments, "These results show that the declarations of glyphosate as the active principle for toxicity are scientifically wrong and that the toxicity assessment is also erroneous: glyphosate is tested for long-term health effects at the regulatory level without its formulants—which are composed of toxic petroleum residues and arsenic. We call for immediate transparency of the formulations and—above all—of any health tests conducted on them. The acceptable levels of glyphosate residues in food and drinks should be divided immediately by a factor of at least one thousand because of these hidden poisons. Glyphosate-based herbicides (amongst other pesticides) should be banned."

> One very important way to triumph over health challenges is to learn the truth about whether the food you consider to be healthy is actually healthy. It takes courage to discover the truth, but the results can be life changing.

Michael Hansen of *Consumer Reports* explained that it was very likely that petroleum-based waste was being added into pesticides as a way to simply discard or "recycle" them and, containing heavy metals and also arsenic, contributed to increasing the toxicity of the products. The petroleum-based chemicals were considered to be inert, and therefore were not tested or proven safe in any way. "There should not be any arsenic in glyphosate-based herbicides," Hansen said. "That much is clear."

In 2017, Moms Across America also tested orange juice and found glyphosate and AMPA residues in all five of the major orange juice brands tested. In researching citrus farming, we learned that copper is often sprayed on the trees to fight fungus. As mentioned previously, copper is an effective spermicide. What if serving a young man a glass of conventional orange juice in the morning is actually sterilizing him?

Also in 2017, the Organic Consumers Association tested and revealed glyphosate in Ben & Jerry's ice cream. Their national campaign to ask them to switch to glyphosate free, organic milk, and other organic ingredients was a success, proving once again the power of the consumers when they have the correct information.

The findings from our urine testing of thirty-six American children released in 2017, which included children who were fed "healthy" (some organic) food. and yet did *not* have lower levels of glyphosate and toxins, suddenly made sense when I reviewed the CFIA results. I discovered that the foods most often used in gluten-free, vegan, and vegetarian foods—which health conscious parents often feed their children *regardless of whether those foods are organic*, were the most highly contaminated with glyphosate residues. This was very disturbing. According to the CFIA test results, the people in America and Canada who are spending extra money to buy "healthy" wheat pita, hummus, vegan soy hot dogs, vegetarian chickpea and bean burgers, red lentil soup, and buckwheat noodles are poisoning themselves with the highest levels of glyphosate residues in America.

Vegan and vegetarian proponents often dismiss the importance of promoting organic. I hope these findings make a difference.

> *I have allergies, had a miscarriage and I have gestational diabetes. One of my children has stomach problems. We are vegetarians, so we do eat very healthy and should not have any of these problems. However, when we stick to all organic, our health concerns seem to go away.* —VICKI J.

I will never forget the conversation my husband and I once had with a supporter. She shared that her daughter was eating "healthy" and did not know why she has had to have three surgeries costing $60,000 each for chronic gut issues. I asked what she ate. She said she was vegan, and was eating whole chickpeas, hummus, lentils, vegetables, soy, and whole wheat bread every day. "Healthy food," she said, but then she admitted it was not organic. I had to hold myself back from groaning. I told her about the glyphosate levels detected by the CFIA, and she gasped. Then she told me that her other daughter was not vegan but was also starting to have gut issues. I asked her if anyone around her used Roundup. She grew silent, then said that her husband sprayed it on the back patio all the time and that the girls walked barefoot out there. My husband and I looked at each other with grief. Needless to say, this woman has since made huge changes which will likely lead to reduced health issues, struggle, and health-care costs. Success over these health issues will not come, however, if one is not curious or willing to ask questions and hear the truth.

From Testing to Proof

We are now able to test for many things—but testing provides knowledge not a cure. Below are testimonials from moms who may or may not have gone to the experts for testing—but either way, they realized they had a problem, went about solving it, and then shared their findings so that others could benefit as well.

> *My son had daily asthma attacks, needed glasses, and was recommended to be held back a year at school. When I found out about GMOs and switched to organic, his asthma disappeared, he no longer needed glasses, and he is now at the top of his class.* —Karen L.
>
> *I have a teenage son who was severely autistic. I found out about GMOs two years ago and went all organic. This was difficult, as I am a single mom making $40,000 a year, but I did it. My father noticed a difference in just two weeks and asked if my son was on a new drug. I said, "Nope, just went all organic." My son entered high school this past fall and not one of his teachers could tell that he ever had autism.* —Cindy S.

> *After my son was diagnosed with autism I quickly realized that it was up to me to figure out how to get him better. Doctors knew so little and they wanted me to drug him. I knew there had to be another way. I wanted to heal the causes, not just mask symptoms or give him dangerous drugs. I wanted to do it naturally. After over a decade of research, trial and error, and more than $100,000 spent, my son today is fully recovered from all his symptoms of anxiety, oppositional defiance, aggression, stomachaches, headaches, and more. I now share exactly what I did for him with other parents to help them get their children better. Children can get better. Mine did. I believe yours can, too.*
>
> —Karen Thomas, author of *Naturally Healing Autism*

These three boys have new futures because their moms found out about GMOs and glyphosate. I say that our country—and maybe even our world—has a new future because their moms found-out about GMOs and glyphosate. Who knows what these three boys will invent or contribute to our society? Think of the inventors of Google and Facebook.

Many women reported that they had health issues, too:

> *I went GMO-free and after about a month, my fibromyalgia went away.* —Belinda M.

> *I have enough proof to keep on doing what I think is best for my family, and that is eliminating GMOs. I had IBS, acid reflux, unexplainable athlete's foot that wouldn't go away, and prediabetes. Once we changed our lifestyle, all these things went away. I share my story with people. I don't know how much more proof they need, but this did it for me. It is a cycle that is killing our earth and humankind for profit. They know what impact GMOs have on the ecosystem, but to them money makes the world go round. Without devastation, there is no profit for them.* —Karina O.

> *Yay for non-GMO diets and organic options! Sixty-four pounds gone! Obesity that I am no longer living with!* —Amberle M.

I had chronic digestive issues, but they soon went away when I switched to an organic whole foods diet. My daughter was diagnosed with ulcerative colitis but keeps it in check with a healthy diet. —Cindy B.

I was diagnosed with gastroesophageal reflux disease and was in a tremendous amount of pain. Tired of taking pills every day to combat the effects of the condition, I decided to research why food was hurting me now, when it never did before. Since switching to GMO-free or organic whenever possible, I have not had to take a single pill. What do you know—the pain is gone! —Colleen G.

Ten years ago, I was diagnosed with breast cancer for the second time. Blood tests revealed I have the BRCA1 gene. My three daughters were tested and two out of three carry the gene. At that time, we asked the geneticist ways to reduce the risk of getting breast cancer, and he said one way was to stay away from GMOs! —Julie J.

Our husbands are being affected as well:

When my husband and I started actively avoiding GMOs in our food, several ailments melted away. But it is increasingly difficult, as more news comes out of more and more GMOs in more and more items. When we cut seriously back on suspect foods, my husband's allergies improved, we both lost weight and my uncomfortable digestive issues have disappeared. —Cindy M.

My husband suffered from GI issues, which have decreased significantly since cutting out GMO products. I took this information to the Rockland County school nurses and was surprised by how many were not aware. —Margaret D.

My husband was told several years ago that he has a "fatty" liver. Since switching to non-GMO and organic foods, my stomach issues are gone and at my husband's last doctor visit, his "fatty" liver has improved. —Colleen C.

> *My husband was in the hospital five times last year. Doctors wanted to remove part of his intestine because it was so infected. Instead, doctors pumped him full of antibiotics for a week and when he got out of the hospital I changed his diet and all our family food choices to non-GMO foods. WOW! What a difference! He's doing great and food never tasted so good! I will march, sign petitions—anything to reclaim our healthy labeled food choices. Godspeed. Just say no to GMOs . . . Moms Across America!* —Rhonda L.

Teachers are confirming the skyrocketing health care crisis in America:

> *I teach music to elementary age children and I work with all the kids in the entire school. These days I get stacks of health sheets on the kids with food allergies, some of them life-threatening. When I started teaching about twenty years ago, I got no such documents.*
> —Julie K.

Reality Check

Historically, in tribal times, men have been the ones to protect and provide. However, women have been the ones to decide what their tribe ate and prolong the longevity of their culture. If mothers did not trust their instinct and fed their tribe poison berries or rotten food, their tribe might perish. In the United States for the past twenty years, however, GMO food has not been labeled, and therefore we have had no way of knowing what is in our food and the health of our nation has declined as a result.

Health in America Today

- Of the top seventeen most developed countries, the USA is last in health, spending the highest amount of money on health care and yet having the lowest rating of health.

- One out of two of children in this country have a chronic illness including autism, allergies, autoimmune disorders, asthma, diabetes, and obesity.

- More than thirty million Americans have diabetes. The increase of diabetes alone will bankrupt the US health-care system in less than a decade if it continues at its present rate.

- One out of two of American males and one out of three females are expected to get cancer. That's two hundred million Americans. Glyphosate has been designated a Class 2 probable carcinogen by the World Health Organization (WHO).

- The CDC reports that the rate of birth defects doubled between 1995 and 2005. Latina women's rates increased as much as 263 percent. From Hawai'i to Washington state to Arkansas, our moms tell us tragic stories of birth defects and miscarriages.

- The USA is number one for infant deaths on day one of life. According to the Save the Children report of 2015, we have 50 percent more infants that die on day one than all other countries in the industrialized world combined. It is a silent crisis. This is too devastating to be in the news or on Facebook, but it is impacting families across America.

- Colitis is up 47 percent and Crohn's disease is up 79 percent in the past ten years. On Facebook, the majority of the Crohn's disease or colitis page posts are from twenty-year-olds. They post that they are getting their intestines sewn up, have colostomy bags, and are in so much pain they go on disability—possibly for the rest of their lives. In addition to the tragic suffering, how is this sustainable for our economy? It's not.

- According to the Liver Foundation, one out of ten Americans now has liver disease. A January 2017 study proved that even very low levels of Roundup caused nonalcoholic fatty liver disease in animals.

- Pesticides are linked to a loss of IQ. The average American's IQ has dropped seven points since the introduction of GMOs. We are literally "dumbing down" America by allowing neurotoxins in our food and water.

- Almost fifty-eight million Americans today have a mental illness. That's one out of five. This includes our pilots on airplanes, politicians, teachers, policemen, doctors, and loved ones. Mental illness impacts a person's potential and the safety of our communities.

Reality Check—Mental Illness, Violence, and Drug Addiction

An article titled "Cereal Killers" in the *Smithsonian Magazine*, February 2018 issue revealed that hamsters in cornfields in France that ate "monoculture, high-yield, corn sprayed with pesticides and herbicides" became cannibals and the mothers ate their young. When the researcher, Mathilde Tissier, Ph.D. candidate at the University of Strasbourg introduced vitamin B3 into their diet, they stopped the cannibalism. She learned that the corn was binding the B3 and niacin, impacting the hamster's behavior. If introducing just one vitamin into an animal's diet can stop violent behavior, how could this practice alter human behavior? What if our children, teens, and other citizens with mental illness or behavioral and learning disorders were tested for vitamin and mineral deficiencies? What if simple dietary changes and supplements could stop at least some of the acts of violence in our nation? In 2018 there were 18 school shootings in just the first six weeks, that's a school shooting every two and a half days. This is a crisis that needs immediate action!

Another crisis America is grappling with is the opioid crisis. Drug addiction is crippling communities across the country. What is missing from this conversation is prevention through healthful eating, especially for our lowest income citizens. Access to fresh organic produce is a necessary investment for our nation's health. Health regulatory agencies must have the courage to enforce laws to make access to whole, organic foods a priority. With access to affordable toxin free and organic food, consumers could prevent some of these tragic addictions by eating healthy and being healthy so they do not feel compelled to take drugs in the first place.

One of the leading reasons drug users start using is depression and chronic pain. Depression and chronic pain have been shown to be linked to pesticides in our food and environment. When glyphosate destroys the beneficial gut bacteria, much of the body's serotonin storage, the body is then unable to feel satiated, satisfied, and will likely become depressed and addicted to substances it normally might not become addicted to. In addition, the depression and serotonin imbalance lead doctors to prescribe selective serotonin reuptake inhibitors (SSRI's) which have been shown to result in higher rates of suicide and homicidal behavior in teens.

Crohn's disease and colitis, stomach disorders which are very painful, have increased exponentially since GMOs and glyphosate have been allowed in our food system. Both diseases are common reasons for doctors to prescribe opioids. Over 60,000 people died of opioid-related deaths in 2017 alone.

Psychotropic drugs, mixed with a deficiency of vitamins and minerals from junk food and toxins in the food, are a dangerous mixture that is likely a leading factor in the mass shootings which are causing untold grief in our nation. In order to stop school shootings and widespread violence, we must look not only at gun laws and more medications, but to the neurotoxins in the food combined with vitamin and mineral deficiencies and drug side effects as well. I assert that a new policy to add vitamin and mineral testing for deficiency and dietary counseling to reduce toxic exposure for all students before entering school would be an important step in restoring health and reducing violence in America.

To summarize, chemical farming, GMOs, and glyphosate herbicides are destroying our gut bacteria and therefore our immune systems, causing organ damage, reproductive harm, compromising our blood-brain barriers and cell formation—all of which lead to the systematic destruction of the potential of our children and the future of America.

However, this alarming information has roused groups of people across the country and around the world to speak up, connect, teach, and support each other . . . creating new communities of caring people who inspire and strengthen our nation.

PART TWO

UNSTOPPABLE COMMUNITY

CHAPTER FOUR
TRUST, TRUTH, AND COMMUNITY

"Never doubt that a small group of thoughtful, committed citizens can change the world. Indeed, it is the only thing that ever has."
—MARGARET MEAD

WHEN I LEARNED about the reality of our toxic food system, lack of government regulation, and risk of harm from the food supply that we thought we could trust not to have hidden dangers, I felt deeply betrayed. I had been lied to—as had all of America. I understood, logically, why the chemical corporations needed to lie to prevent lawsuits and protect their profits. But understanding it did not ease the sting of betrayal. Not only did I lose my sense of trust in both the government and food manufacturers, but I also had trouble trusting even my own judgment for a while. I experienced a crisis of trust—feeling isolated, unsafe, and lonely. It wasn't until I began to meet other people who knew what was going on that I began to feel hope and trust again.

I used to think of the word "community" in the same context as the word "taxes." It was something I put up with. People were generally annoying. There were a few good ones, but most of the time, I just wanted to be left alone to live my life the way I wanted to.

Then my kids got sick. I reached out and quickly connected to new groups of people interested in helping who had no agendas. They only wanted to offer the truth as they experienced it. They were from all over the country—in fact, from all over the world. They were my newfound community of social media contacts. I had found my enthusiastic team, my committed contingency, and I was able to learn from farmers, scientists, teachers, health coaches, journalists, activists, politicians, lawyers, students, and doctors that I would otherwise have never met. As my online community expanded, they supported me in getting more connected to what the internet calls my "in real life" community. I felt empowered to venture out to a local meeting about GMOs . . . and that is where I found greater connection, inspiration, appreciation, and empowerment. Connecting with my community meant that I found other people who agreed with my intuition to protect my children. I found people who shared similar stories and confirmed my suspicions. I began to trust myself again.

Once I got involved locally and began sharing the truth, I decided to take on being a public speaker on the subject of GMOs. I wanted nothing more than for people to learn the truth about GMOs and empower them to take action. I felt compelled. I made up a business card that said "speaker" on it, and within a few months I was asked to speak at a wellness expo. Not long after that, I was asked to speak for various groups across the country. It was—and still is—a great honor, and I am always thrilled with what I learn from others when I attend an event.

One of the best community gatherings of parents struggling with health, learning, and behavioral issues with their children is the annual AutismOne conference. I would venture to say that 98% percent of the attendees are mothers. Often held in Chicago, over 200 speakers and companies with health products converge to present new science and possible solutions to the public. At the first conference I attended as a speaker, Dr. Stephanie Seneff and I were two of the few, if not the only, people focusing on GMOs and glyphosate in connection with autism. The next year, almost every speaker who discussed detoxing and health improvements mentioned GMOs and glyphosate. Word travels fast in our communities. Moms talk. We share solutions. Gathering together and sharing the truth—not whitewashed by corporate agendas, not made pretty or dumbed down—empowers mothers enormously.

The following is just one of the examples of the incredibly intelligent, committed, and resourceful moms from the community that I met at AutismOne.

So Many of Our Kids

"ADHD, and Autism are not "Psychiatric Disorders" that warrant large doses of medication. They are actually metabolic, immunologic, and neurologic digestive disorders that require a biomedical protocol."
—THE AMERICAN HOLISTIC MEDICAL ASSOCIATION

Jennifer Giustra-Kozek is a board-certified psychotherapist, speaker, and author of *Healing without Hurting: Treating ADHD, Apraxia, and Autism Spectrum Disorders Naturally & Effectively without Harmful Medication*. Here is Jennifer's story in her own words:

Things I Learned While Trying to Heal My Child from Autism, Apraxia, Anxiety, and ADHD

By practice, I'm a psychotherapist who has been working for over a decade in the world of mainstream medicine. I have a body of experience that has allowed me to develop a strong understanding of both medicine's strengths and its weaknesses. But beyond my work, I'm also a mom who fiercely loves her children. For their sakes, when it comes to their health, I've always explored all available options—an approach that I'm proud to say has led me to find far better solutions than any conventional specialist had ever offered.

My work has allowed me to cross paths with a seemingly endless number of psychiatrists and general practitioners who, for the most part, have one thing in common. They all see medication as the optimal form of treatment for the vast majority of what they diagnose as being attention deficit hyperactivity disorder (ADHD), anxiety, sleep issues, depression, and obsessive-compulsive disorder.

For a long time, I wondered about the cavalier prescribing of drugs but bit my tongue. Who was I to question physicians who had the benefit of many more years of medical training than I had? My viewpoint changed in 2006 after I had a child who suffered similar health challenges.

I knew doctors would recommend medication. I also knew I

didn't want my son to go down that road for fear it would severely damage his lively, beautiful spirit.

As my husband, Steve, and I tried to make do with physical and behavioral therapies, I read many medical journal articles about the link between autism, mental health issues, and toxins causing epigenetic changes in our DNA. I also learned that malnutrition, food sensitivities, viral infections, intestinal permeability, immune system issues, metabolic issues, and digestive issues also play a role. These discoveries led us to realize that these disorders could be real medical illnesses treatable with natural remedies that didn't involve intrusive, personality-altering medication. While we were skeptical at first, the potential rewards were so great that these methods outside the mainstream seemed well worth trying. And I am happy that we did! Addressing and treating the underlying pathologies of ADHD and autism lead to marked improvements in my son, Evan—without the side effects of medication.

I learned that our emotions are primarily governed by the state of our immune and intestinal systems. Interesting fact: there are more neurons lining the digestive tract than in either the peripheral nervous system or the spinal column. This "second brain" is known as the enteric nervous system that controls the function of the gastrointestinal tract. Dr. Michael Gershon, chairman of the Department of Anatomy and Cell Biology at New York–Presbyterian Hospital/Columbia University Medical Center, an expert in the nascent field of neuro-gastroenterology, explains that 90 percent of the fibers of the vagus nerve in the neck carry information from the gut to the brain, and not the other way around. Interestingly, 95 percent of the body's serotonin is in the bowels. Also, research suggests that there is an essential relationship between the gut microbiome and the development and function of the brain and nervous system. Diet plays a critical role in the establishment, maturation, and maintenance of microbial diversity in the gut ecosystem that is crucial for a healthy brain. Also, glyphosate used in GMO farming not only introduces highly toxic chemicals into our bodies, it negatively impacts our friendly gut bacteria and favors the growth of harmful bacteria.

Our Healing Story

We removed all processed food, pesticides, and foods containing genetically modified ingredients. We also eliminated all foods Evan was either moderately or highly sensitive to including dairy, gluten, and egg. We healed his gut with medicinal herbs and used some gentle detox homeopathy remedies. We started balancing Evan nutritionally by introducing more wholesome organic food, which he welcomed more easily once we healed his upset intestinal system.

After changing our dietary lifestyle and seeking help from functional medicine MDs and naturopathic doctors the progress we began to see was nothing short of astounding. Within a few months, we started to see significant improvements in social behavior, speech, mood, and attention.

We then identified Evan's genetic mutations and adjusted his diet accordingly. The MTHFR gene mutation was affecting how he metabolized vitamin B12 to folate/folic acid correctly. Pyroluria is a mutation that affects our important brain nutrients, zinc, and vitamin B6. He also had the COMT gene mutation that affected how he metabolized amino acids effectively. This mutation could adversely affect the creation and balancing of hormones/neurotransmitters.

We also started taking advantage of brain training therapies like neurofeedback, vision therapy, and brain gym activities to help integrate his senses and reflexes. We also did many Eastern medicine therapies and treatments such as acupuncture and energy healing. I discovered that over the course of treatment, Evan started improving exponentially in all areas of development—including emotionally, socially, physically, and academically.

We now saw a confident boy who was eager to join group activities and was more independent in daily activities of living. His motor skills jumped up from extremely disordered to barely noticeable and he is now on the basketball team at his mainstream school.

So, we continue the appointments with our holistic physicians to address any emerging health concerns or imbalances. We continue his dietary modifications to optimize his health and keep up with therapies so that he can be 100 percent capable of fulfilling his potential.

The Silent Community

Many of our communities do not come together out of joy, but out of grief. Almost all women who have miscarried have experienced the profound anger, sadness, and sometimes guilt and shame that accompany such an extreme loss. And there are more and more of us having this life-altering experience. Where there were once four fertility clinics in a county such as Orange County, California, there are now fourteen. I recently met an in vitro fertilization (IVF) center owner who boasted that his industry expected a 22 percent growth per year for the next twenty years. I was horrified. It is time we share and are open to learning about our new reality.

Young couples today who have been married for a few years might wince if Aunt Annie asks them if they are going to have kids. Mothers of one child might cringe at a question about having more. Couples who have two boys might be suppressing tears of anguish if Grandma asks them if they want to have a girl. Too many couples have experienced multiple miscarriages and are hiding their pain.

When I learned about GMOs in 2012 and later more about glyphosate, the issue that concerned me the most was that when rats were fed GMOs, they experienced reproductive harm and the third generation was completely sterile. Infertility, miscarriages, and stillborn infants are particularly devastating. A study by S. Parvez et al. released in March 2018 showed that maternal exposure to glyphosate led to a significant increase in shortened gestation of the pregnancy. Shortened gestation means not only a premature birth, with probable developmental delays, but could also mean a miscarriage or infant death. There is no way to return an infant who has been lost in this way to a mother. The loss of life isolates us and can divide households and end marriages. It also has long-term effects on society as a whole.

I know just how devastating this situation is firsthand. It is not something I ever talk about in my speeches or in my interviews. Only once or twice have I shared this when it seemed particularly timely. Like many of my friends and family members, I also had a miscarriage and lost the life of our child. I was in the second month of the pregnancy, so I was not showing yet, but a loss of one's child at any stage of development is indescribably painful. My intuition says it was a girl—the girl I will never be able to watch grow up and perhaps become a mother herself someday. This loss dulls the joy in my life in very unexpected and subtle ways.

I will see bows and hair ties for sale in a pharmacy by the nail polish and suddenly want to cry. I watch a paper towel commercial with a girl hugging her mother and I mourn. I can be perfectly content with my life, my boys, and my marriage, but still the loss and sadness for what I will never experience runs so deep and is so palpable that silence seems to be the only form of expression that helps me keep it together.

Within a year of losing our baby, I did conceive again. I am fortunate to have three healthy boys. I am forever grateful for the gift of life that they are to me.

I can only imagine the grief of the women in the world who have lost multiple babies or who have never conceived at all. I can only imagine the pain of carrying a baby to full term, giving birth to what you would expect to be a live, healthy baby, and then experiencing loss. It is soul crushing. It can leave a woman feeling like she has been scooped out like a pumpkin and all that is left is a paper thin shell. Or it can leave her feeling heavier than a thousand planets—dead and dense and dark inside.

I grieve with all of you. I insist that you do not blame yourselves. We may never know what caused these miscarriages. It could have been the Roundup that the landscaper sprayed on the sidewalks and condo community property or it could have been the GMO soy milk we drank to avoid dairy. It could have been a deformity that just randomly occurred due to a thousand chemical reactions happening in every moment in our bodies. We will never know. Not knowing still haunts me.

Hidden Agendas

While not knowing can be painful, it can also be very motivating. The lack of knowledge in young women, mothers-to-be, and the community in general about the endocrine disrupting capabilities of glyphosate and many chemicals in our food, water, plastics, household furniture, and even pajamas spurs me to keep going and telling others about the risks.

Some people use the "not knowing" as a cop-out for not taking responsibility. Alison L. Van Eenennaam, Ph.D., cooperative extension specialist in animal genomics and biotechnology at U.C. Davis Department of Animal Science and former Monsanto employee who was featured in the pro-GMO movie *Food Evolution,* used her own miscarriage to shame activists like me for "using a tragedy to promote their agenda," apparently failing to realize that she herself was doing exactly what she accused us of doing.

The difference between her agenda and mine is that if you follow her advice—to just accept that you will never know what caused your miscarriage because "some things don't have a cause"—then you will likely continue to expose yourself to potentially harmful chemicals. If you follow the precautionary principle (the principle that the introduction of a new product or process whose ultimate effects are disputed or unknown should be resisted) instead, the only consequence is that you would be paying a bit more upfront for organic food (but saving a lot more in doctor's bills later). In addition, you would most likely avoid potentially endocrine disrupting chemicals and reduce the risk of harm to your fetus. You might even save your baby's life. You will never know what harm or disease your family avoided. I prefer that kind of not knowing.

Some people do know. One young couple told me, "Many of our friends have decided not to get pregnant because they think their bodies are too toxic. They feel that their bodies are not safe." How tragic. It's one thing to not feel safe in a certain city or job, because you can move or quit. It's another thing entirely to feel that your own body is unsafe. This is unacceptable.

In summer of 2017, the judge presiding over the lawsuit by Baum, Hedlund, Aristei & Goldman, with Robert F. Kennedy, Jr., representing nearly a thousand plaintiffs whose family members handled Roundup and subsequently died of, or were affected by, non-Hodgkin lymphoma, released Monsanto's documents to the public. Carey Gillam, veteran journalist from the nonprofit organization US Right To Know and the author of *Whitewash: The Story of a Weed Killer, Cancer, and the Corruption of Science,* stated that these "documents prompted a wave of outrage for what they revealed: questionable research practices by Monsanto, cozy ties to a top official within the US Environmental Protection Agency, and indications that Monsanto may have engaged in 'ghostwriting' of research studies that appeared to be independent of the company."

Robert F. Kennedy, Jr. (president of Water Keepers Alliance who is working with the law firm of Baum, Hedlund, Aristei & Goldman in Roundup cancer lawsuits against Monsanto,) shared with me the following for this book:

Monsanto executives knew that Roundup was causing cancer and other injuries to its customers and consumers for decades. Following the playbook, they developed plans to defend their other toxic products like PCBs and Agent Orange. Monsanto lied to the public, subverted regulators, purchased sciences, and corrupted public officials to milk profits from poison.

These documents also uncovered a tragic decision by Monsanto's lead toxicologist Donna Farmer. In a 2012 document that she edited regarding a scientific study on male rats exposed to glyphosate, she changed a sentence that originally read, "Although the results suggested, they fail to confirm that glyphosate causes miscarriages." She revised it to say, "The results fail to confirm that glyphosate causes miscarriages." The latter sentence is very different from the former. This action taken by Donna Farmer was not only a betrayal of both the scientific community and humanity at large, it removes the ability of the readers—whether they be other scientists, regulatory agencies, farmers, or consumers who may wish to use glyphosate herbicides—to be fully informed of the potential risks. The fact that the results from this one study, which suggested glyphosate's potential to cause miscarriages, was hidden from the public and government agencies clearly shows Monsanto's determination to continue to sell their products at any cost.

I met Donna Farmer on two occasions—once at a Monsanto shareholders' meeting, and once at the glyphosate hearing at the California EPA's Office of Environmental Health Hazard Assessment (OEHHA). Each time, it was clear that she was feigning interest in the studies I presented. She pretended to not remember me from one time to the next, and never directly answered my questions—especially the ones about glyphosate being found in vaccines and her own admission that Monsanto's study showed that glyphosate caused harm when it was injected into animals. Apparently, I was not the only one who had these difficulties when attempting to communicate with her. After her attempts to protect the reputation of Monsanto and cover up the dangers of glyphosate herbicides revealed in the legal papers were made public, she was also exposed in November 2017 on the television show *The Doctors* in front of millions of viewers. She has not made any public statement since then about glyphosate being injected into animals. As any mother will tell you, *It never pays to hide the truth—the truth always comes out.* And when it does, it hardly seems worth it—no amount of money can buy you a better reputation.

Trusting Farmers, Trusting Nature

The family farm community is the epicenter of the organic food movement. Meeting honest, caring, hardworking farmers and learning the truth about their work has been one of the biggest blessings of being involved in this cause. The farmers I have met care not just about feeding people, their livelihood and family, but also about the land . . . protecting the soil for generations to come.

Monsanto claims to be a "sustainable agriculture company," which means, according to Merriam-Webster Dictionary, *relating to, or being a method of harvesting or using a resource so that the resource is not depleted or permanently damaged.* Nothing could be further from the truth. The products that Monsanto sells—herbicides—have been proven to deplete and harm the soil for decades, pollute the water, damage and diminish our resources of clean water and food. Furthermore, by taking seeds that exist in nature, genetically altering and patenting them, then charging up to 30 percent more each year for the "technology" that usually causes the seeds to tolerate herbicides, they are actually entrapping farmers into their cycle of chemical sales. When Monsanto merges with Bayer as planned, they will monopolize 70 percent of the cottonseed market, and higher prices will be inevitable. They only thing that GMO chemical companies hope to sustain is their profits. Their hidden agenda and deceit have not gone unnoticed by many farmers, however, who have switched and forged ahead without GMOs and toxic chemicals.

In the process of communicating the dangers of GMOs and related chemicals, I have had the privilege to meet extraordinary people, whom I otherwise never would have met, who are working in very specific areas to transform the food supply. I met salt of the earth farmer Pat Trask in South Dakota, who went all the way to the supreme court to prevent GMO alfalfa from being allowed in the animal feed supply because, "When I learned that there would be one company [Monsanto] that wanted control over all of the seed, I thought, them's fightin' words." Farmers like Trask resist GMOs not just because of the control over the seed supply, and not just because they are being forced to buy their seeds from one company and not replant their own seeds, but because they fundamentally disagree with a chemical company altering life as God made it. They are deeply religious people and believe that "when God created life, and said it was good, it was." They see it as blasphemous to alter life, patent it, and then sell it as a commodity.

I met Howard Vlieger, a farmer from Iowa, thanks to Kathleen Hallal of Irvine, California. A busy mom of three boys, Kathleen still managed to arrange for Howard to speak about GMOs and toxins in Southern California fourteen times in just six days. She was—and still is—a mother on a mission. Since supporting the start of Moms Across America, she and a dedicated group of parents have formed the advocacy group Non-Toxic Communities, had the city of Irvine discontinue the use of toxic chemicals such as glyphosate, and inspired many other counties to switch to organic practices as well. Moms and farmers are connecting and spreading the word. Because I was able to meet Howard Vlieger and attend his talks so many times, I gained a strong foundation of knowledge about farming, the confidence to speak publicly about the topic, a deep respect for farmers, and a lifelong friend.

Howard regards his position as a self-described "student of the soil" with great reverence. He states, "It is an amazing opportunity to be a caretaker of the soil. The good Lord made an amazing creation when He created the soil. It is a true joy to continue the never-ending learning experience of working with all the biological and elemental components of the soil to produce clean, high-quality, nutritious food for all families to eat. It is an even greater privilege to work with family farmers to help them gain a better understanding of crop and livestock production to produce premium quality food nature's way."

His perspective—along with the dedication of moms like Kathleen and the hundreds of thousands of people who now support Moms Across America, who are willing to pay for quality food—could literally transform the farming industry and health of our country. We just need conventional farmers to see that pathway as well.

It was with great relief that I learned in the fall of 2017 through Howard at the Heirloom Expo in Santa Rosa, California, that a nontoxic alternative to Roundup has been developed. Using it will be an essential part of being able to shift away from toxic chemical farming and landscaping.

Another dedicated individual is Bob Streit, Ph.D., a delightful farmer and educator from Iowa with a twinkle in his blue eyes who works enthusiastically and courageously, nationally and abroad, to bring alternatives to farmers who feel trapped in the toxic treadmill of chemical cocktails. Bob is on the front lines of transforming the food supply. His only weapons are a big heart, honesty, and farming innovations that work with nature instead of against it.

Farmer Bob Streit contributes the following insights on the state of farming around the world:

At present, there seems to be a big shift globally as to how aware farmers are of how dangerous different pesticides are to human health. In most European countries, the people purchasing the food tend to rely more on small markets, where they meet the growers and see the crops in the fields. They prefer fresh food where much of it is grown, raised, or caught locally. What might make both European consumers and producers different from us is that they identify with top quality food. They are able to read the many research articles on the effect of today's pesticides on human health. Not as many of their media outlets and politicians try to hush up the use and effects of pesticides and fertilizers that pose harm to the human population and their animals.

I have made thirteen trips to South America to work with local farmers to reduce chemical usage and resist crop damage. I am on the USDA soybean rust task force with other farmers and scientists. That is the worst crop disease possible and will eventually threaten the world's protein supply. We work with the top scientists in Brazil, Argentina, Uruguay, and Paraguay. These scientists are also very up-to-date on the research that has been done because they often know the schools or people doing the research personally.

In Brazil and Argentina, they love their beef, and people in those countries know it comes from ranches and pastures, not the supermarkets. Fresh fruit and vegetables are ever present due to those countries' warmer climates and year-round production. The Brazilians and Argentinians treat meals and eating together as part of their social fabric. Food is something to be enjoyed and treasured.

Currently in South America, the citizen's level of awareness to the health effects of some of the herbicides and insecticides is very high. There are different economic castes and the poorer people often squat or rent in rural areas that are interspersed with fields that get sprayed by plane or custom applicators. The wealthier landowners, however, don't know many of their neighbors (who are spraying) and often are not very aware of the exposure problems or dismiss it as part of the cost of living in a high disease and high insect part of the world. Therefore, the landowners do nothing.

A high percentage of the residents have access to the medical reports that tell of the consequence of pesticide usage. There are many prominent physicians and researchers who are doing good work and make sure the population is educated on the issues. Those people are very willing to protest corporations they see as evil and act like their lives depend on it. As for the landowners, even the larger farmers recognize that they have to work more with nature than try to get it to bend to their needs. This means that conservation buffers of 20 percent up to 80 percent are required in some areas. They recognize that every living creature exists for a purpose.

Around the world, more growers are looking around them and realizing that they are trapped in an escalating battle with weeds and insects and the modern modified crops are no longer delivering on their promises. There are many forty-year-old and under producers who are more willing to study plant nutrition and address the plants' nutritional needs rather than just blindly follow self-serving advice from an industry-funded spokesperson.

Five years ago, there were very few farmers mentioning soil health or regenerative agriculture. Today, those are very popular topics at field days and technology fairs around the world. More producers and agriculture professionals know that good healthy soil is a gift that must be protected and are helping to educate new converts. The same crowds are now hearing more about the connection between pesticides and some of their production practices and want to make a difference on the positive side. They recognize that their kids and grandkids are also being affected.

I would say that 75 to 80 percent of my farmers ask me about the chemicals and whether I know the facts and if I can give them any information. They recognize they have attended too many funerals for family, friends, or neighbors. I personally have had eleven family members afflicted with cancer. Two-thirds of them have not made it.

Farmers who raise animals are being affected by GMOs and glyphosate as well. Ib Pedersen, a pig farmer from Denmark who coauthored a pig study with German scientist Monika Kruger that showed a higher level of birth defects and miscarriages in sows that ate grains that had been sprayed with glyphosate, stated:

> Any farmer who switches away from GMOs and Roundup will experience improved health in their herd and crops.
>
> I know of the scientific studies on malformations due to the chemical Roundup. I know that one in eighty people in certain towns in Argentina have the same birth defects after being exposed to the chemical. And I know of fourteen Danish people born with deformities of the same type.
>
> Now, what I have seen in my pigs makes me wonder what we are doing—not just to them, but to ourselves. And it scares me.
>
> A farmer's task is to provide nutritious and healthy food for consumers. GMOs and Roundup provide neither. We can look back to DDT and how we once thought that was healthy. That should remind us that we cannot ignore the warning signs for glyphosate.

Scientist and farmer Dr. Don Huber, professor emeritus of plant pathology at Perdue University also warns us, "future historians may well look back upon our time and write, not about how many pounds of pesticide we did or did not apply, but how willing we were to sacrifice our children and jeopardize future generations with this massive experiment we call genetic engineering that is based on flawed science and failed promises just to benefit the bottom line of a commercial enterprise."

Scientists Speaking the Truth

The scientific community plays a crucial role in progress. However, a problem arises when new science is automatically perceived as being progress without care having been paid to scientific integrity.

There is much talk about science in the news . . . believing in it, science being real . . . people marching "for science." I find this language purposely vague and manipulative. For science . . . which science? The science paid for by the chemical companies that stand to profit from the results? Or the science conducted by independent scientists that debunks the claims of the corporations? Which scientists should we trust?

After having done research for years, and spoken with experts who have researched for decades, I tend to trust the scientists who see the actual reality, no matter how damning it is for them or for the corporate funders of their universities. They want to share the truth. They do not try to belittle our food movement by referring to mothers as emotional and they do not scoff at us when we take to the podium. They respect women and mothers. They believe that we can—and are—making a difference. In fact, many of them have been inspired by our movement, raised funds for testing, and have conducted serious scientific studies—because of us mothers speaking out about our concerns.

But I don't just trust certain scientists because I agree with their findings and their findings support what we suspect. I trust certain scientists because of the risk they are willing to take to warn us of possible harm that we can then avoid. I trust the scientists who are willing to go against the current corrupt system and expose the lack of integrity of both certain corporations and parts of the government. The EPA is currently a huge contributor to the corruption in our food system. There are few who have seen the inner workings of the EPA who are willing to come forward. Evaggelos Vallianatos, Ph.D., who worked at the EPA for decades and is the author of *Poison Spring*, is one of them. He contributed the following for this book:

> I was one of those insiders. It did not take me long to challenge the fake science of regulation. I figured out that, with some exceptions, the EPA brass was at peace with business as usual. Which is to say, these senior managers did not feel uncomfortable with polluted air, water, and food. They probably saw themselves as guardians of the existing corporate economy. EPA scientists and the EPA library had evidence of harm, but the EPA managers did not want to see or act on that evidence.
>
> The EPA has been ignoring its mission because it is in collusion with the industry, such as the manufacturers and merchants of farm sprays. These sprays are biocides—chemicals designed to kill all life. They cripple and kill innumerable species of animals and plants. These poisons also contaminate our food, drinking water, and air. In fact, they are so pervasive in the environment that they poison mothers' breast milk.
>
> I attended meetings where scientists and managers made pol-

icy or discussed important issues. I met with certain of my colleagues for lunch or in their offices and talked about their work and experience. A number of those scientists not only talked to me extensively about the problems they faced within their organization, but also handed me hundreds of key documents illustrating the reasons for their discontent. I read those documents, which included thousands of memoranda, issue papers, briefings, letters, studies, and reports detailing the vast panorama of the EPA's pesticides swamp.

Each individual document might contain a hint or a fact about the intricate and complicated world of pseudoscience camouflaging the steady pollution of this country's food, drinking water, and the rest of the natural world. The major culprits included virulent insect poisons, other bug sprays, and weed killers. Following the trails developed through the web of those hints and facts, I began to grasp the magnitude and seriousness of what lay behind the external, scientifically correct appearance of the pesticides bureaucracy of the EPA.

With each new discovery, I became more determined to reveal the hidden politics of America's poison spring, continuing on the path of Rachel Carson, who summarized in 1962 what was known about the ecological effects of the farmers' sprays. But here I was, decades after Rachel Carson, observing how silent and poison springs come into being, and for whose benefit.

The EPA looks at a chemical's risks to humans and nature, and the conclusions of that investigation make up "risk assessment." But the pesticides law says that the EPA also has to evaluate the "benefits" of that same chemical. At the end of that process, it is up to the EPA administrator to balance the risks and benefits in his or her decision.

In other words, in the best of circumstances, the EPA administrator ought to have enough information about the risks and benefits of a chemical so that he or she can say the risks in this case so exceed the benefits that we must cancel this pesticide, or the benefits of this spray are so great we must keep it on the market while we minimize its threat to people and nature. Who would disagree with such a reasonable process? In actual practice, however, these things are neither reasonable, nor do they happen this way at all.

Not only is the "risk assessment" full of corrupt scientific and political practices, but the "benefits analysis" is just as loaded with pseudoscience and unreliable data so that the "benefits" always look good.

As well as Dr. Vallianatos, former EPA toxicologist Marion Copley was another scientist who took the risk of speaking up. She worked for thirty years researching the effects of chemicals on mice and she repeatedly warned her peers of the danger of glyphosate. In March 2013, as she was dying of breast cancer, Copley wrote a notable letter to Jess Rowland, who was the deputy director of the EPA's pesticide division and head of the Cancer Assessment Review Committee that was evaluating glyphosate. Copley was also serving on the committee. In a letter revealed to the public after her death, she clearly described how glyphosate played a role in the formation of tumors in humans. She named over a dozen specific methods by which it could do the job. "Any one of these mechanisms alone . . . can cause tumors, but glyphosate causes all of them simultaneously," she wrote. "It is essentially certain that glyphosate causes cancer." She specifically said, "Jess: For once in your life, listen to me and don't play your political conniving games with the science to favor the registrants." But he continued to play games, and was even caught writing in an email, regarding the glyphosate assessment, "If I can squash this, I should get a medal." Copley's letter was dated March 2013, a full year before Moms Across America exposed glyphosate in breast milk and met with the EPA, where they stared at us blankly while we admonished them for not protecting Americans from the harm of glyphosate.

Moms and Science—Bring It On!

The community of mothers has grown to be so formidable that we are recognized as one of the biggest problems for the GMO and chemical industry. Being a mother or parent can bring with it a special motivation to seek out the science to support our offsprings' health. When I was interviewed by a Chinese talk show host, Mr. Cui, for a documentary on GMOs, he said, "Monsanto has turned moms into scientists." Being a mother does not mean we cannot comprehend the science and debate with the best of them. We have the science to back us up, so bring it on!

It was November 6, 2014, when I drove to Riverside, California, to debate Professor Brian A. Federici, Ph.D., a scientist and one of the inventors of the Bt toxin GMO. I was fully prepared for the misleading statements I was about to face . . . and I was not surprised by them.

In the debate, Federici continually repeated that there are hundreds of tests showing that GMOs are safe, and that GMOs are needed to feed the world. What he either didn't understand—or refused to admit—was that most of what he was basing his assertions on was simply not true. GMOs have been shown to be harmful in animal studies. We do not need GMO mono crops grown with toxic chemicals to feed the world—we need organic, regenerative agriculture. Studies show that GMO foods are significantly different from non-GMO foods: they have higher levels of synthetic chemicals and some create higher levels of toxins called putrescine and cadaverine and have been shown to cause organ damage in animals.

He spoke of how Bacillus thuringiensis (Bt) toxin corn is made, how the Bt bacteria is harvested from the carcasses of dead grain caterpillars, and how we eat it plentifully in both our GMO and organic food. What he had failed to acknowledge is that the Bt toxin used in organic food is not genetically modified to constantly reproduce more toxins. Instead, it dries up and loses potency in a matter of hours. He asserted that correlation does not equal causation as if that should negate the precautionary principle and we should just go ahead and risk potential harm despite the more than 99 percent correlation between glyphosate and many serious diseases.

Federici had a slide comparing me to a male World Food Prize Nobel Laureate, trying to cast doubt on my intelligence. I have often experienced condescending and dismissive remarks that accuse me of being emotional, antiscience, and fear mongering. Many women in our movement experience the same, and it is obvious to us that sexism is playing a major part in the opposition's tactics. In fact, it has been revealed through disclosure for a lawsuit that Monsanto paid internet trolls to discredit people like me for speaking up about the dangers of Roundup. The troll's attacks were vulgar, misogynistic, and completely false. This behavior not only damages the reputation of truthful people but also fuels the courage of people who honestly believe that Roundup and GMOs are safe. The trolls attack people who are effective in raising awareness. Their presence shows that we are a force to be reckoned with. I think the fact that I am a mother and not a scientist just goes to show that anyone can understand that the technology and motivation behind GMOs are not in the best interest of our health.

When it was my turn to speak, I explained that the foundation of GMO technology is twenty years old. How many of you have a twenty-year-old cell phone? This science is based on the concept that when a scientist inserts foreign protein into the DNA of a completely unrelated species, it will only impact or change that one chain of DNA. This is simply an assumption and is not based on fact. In 2013, Washington University professor John Stamatoyannopoulos discovered that DNA has a double helix, so any alteration to one chromosome of the DNA can and will impact other proteins in the double helix. The changes in the DNA also communicate with the proteins, cells, and DNA around it . . . much like an ecosystem.

A drop of water impacts the air around it, the soil, the plant life, and the birds. Life is not isolated—it is communal. Any changes to one life form impact all life forms. This can be seen in nature by watching the fascinating four-minute video, "How Wolves Change Rivers," on YouTube that shows how the reintroduction of wolves into Yellowstone impacts the migration pattern of the deer, therefore the growth of vegetation, wildlife proliferation, and even the shape of the rivers themselves. For a scientist to think that they can introduce the DNA of one species into another, completely unrelated species and not have it cause havoc within the life form is flawed science and it is simply not in accordance with how nature works.

The GMO scientist's occupation consists of manipulating and attempting to control nature. I believe this involves a fascination with power. Often, people who wish to assert power in a certain area are willing to take risks beyond consideration of health and morality. Take, for example, a book titled *Bold: How to Go Big, Create Wealth, and Impact the World*, by Peter H. Diamandis, which describes how a well-respected CEO of a major corporation would often show up to board meetings with a T-shirt that read "Safety Last." In the name of innovation, progress, success, and profits, corporations will far too often disregard health and safety—and require that their scientists support their choices.

Some believe that GMO scientists are trying to find another way to "solve the problem" of pests and weeds for farmers. Perhaps the real problem is not that bugs and weeds exist. The real problem is that chemical companies think it's their job to solve that problem. It's not. Making chemicals that are safe and useful is their job. GMO scientists and chemical companies never should have tampered with the food system—it should have been left to the farmers. Trapping farmers in a cycle of paying higher prices for GMO seed technology and chemicals is another form of serfdom. The problem is not about bugs and weeds—it's about chemical companies trying to take control of the farmers' domain.

GMO chemical companies do not market themselves as bug and weed killers. They claim that they have taken on the enormous and noble task of "feeding the world." However, the difficulty of feeding the world is also not their problem to solve. Food shortage is not the problem—we waste 40 percent of our food in America, and over 40 percent of us are obese. Worldwide, more people are obese than starving. People with food shortages have a lack of both resources and access to healthy, non-GMO, and organic food and eat cheap, toxic GMO junk food instead. Lack of education, jobs, and distribution of food is the problem. Chemical companies know that what they are doing is causing harm to people. The fact they are continuing those practices is the problem—and is one that they can actually fix.

Many also see a stark difference in the way the genders view these problems. As stated by Dr. Vandana Shiva, "Women do not grow food for profit. They grow food to nurture. This means that the way women grow food will be very different from that of a man who grows food for profit."

Historically, women have been the ones to gather and work with nature. They were the ones responsible to see the signs of changes in the season, to preserve and store food, to save scraps for compost, to grow organic food with combination crops, which keep pests away, and to save the seeds and reuse them the next year. Women, typically, have been the ones in charge of the health of their tribes as well. For women, growing and preparing food and maintaining the good health of the family are inextricably intertwined.

Farmer, national speaker, and educator Dr. Michael McNeill told me recently that when he held a seminar to educate farmers about the dangers of GMOs and Roundup, at first, he had no agreement. The farmers wanted to keep doing things the way they were doing them, which was apparently "easier" than what he was suggesting. But then he held another seminar where he invited the farmers to bring their wives and have lunch. During that seminar, when he spoke of the dangers of glyphosate and Roundup, he saw the wives elbowing their husbands, and whispering, "You are going to do this." That year he had a 90 percent conversion rate of farmers switching from using Roundup to biodiverse farming. It was the women who pushed for the change because they think long-term about health. Trying to take advantage of this situation, Monsanto has initiated Mom Farmer awards, paid mom bloggers to visit their facility and write about the virtues of GMOs, and has supported women who attack GMO skeptics. They know the power of women.

In the debate with Federici, I encouraged the audience by saying that it is MOMS who buy 85 percent of the food. *We* have the power. If we don't buy it, they can't sell it. The Dalai Lama says, "Western women will change the world." Western women are just the start. We need to change the world—all women, from everywhere, together. The time has come to stop listening to the lies being fed to us by scientists who are funded by six major chemical companies and start listening to the millions of mothers who have sick children that are getting better when they get off GMOs.

I addressed the Bt toxin claims of safety by sharing how when Gottfried Glöckner from Germany reported that his cows had gotten Clostridia and many died when they ate GMO Bt corn, he was imprisoned for eighteen months for a made-up crime with funding for the accuser coming from Syngenta lawyers. In addition, the Bt that he mentioned that is in the GMO corn is not the same Bt that is found in organic soil or dead grain larvae. This GMO Bt is genetically engineered to constantly reproduce more toxin, so every cell of the plant becomes, in effect, a Bt factory, which causes holes to form in the bug's stomach when it eats the corn, leading to its death.

When Federici said that the accounts from moms about their children's health improving are all anecdotal, I said "Yes. Our accounts from over one thousand moms are anecdotal, and they are also *our reality*. Our moms have no special interest other than the well-being of their families. They are not paid by organic companies. They have better things to do than to take down biotech. Moms have to tend to homework, soccer practice, doctor appointments, and family budgeting. We would much rather be playing with our toddlers or even cleaning a toilet than poring over scientific studies about the shikimate pathways and how glyphosate destroys them in insects and in humans."

Federici admitted that no one could ever really say whether or not GMOs or pesticides are safe because they are not allowed to do human testing. It is not considered ethical. I pointed out that if it is not considered ethical to test pesticides *on* humans, then it is not ethical to allow pesticides *in* humans through our food supply. The room broke out in thunderous applause.

> No matter what your circumstances—when facing a CEO of a huge company, a scientist of high regard, an intimidating politician, a single adversary, or a massive crowd—be present to, meaning focus on—the love you have for your family. Get that the role you play representing others is more important than any concerns you may have about yourself and you will be clear, strong, and state the truth in a compelling manner. As Zoe Swartz, the leader of Moms Across America's Pennsylvania chapter, said, "A chemical company's right to make a profit in no way surpasses a mother's right to protect her child." Own your right to protect life. Speak up. No matter what.

CHAPTER FIVE
A HEALTHY COMMUNITY STARTS WITH A HEALTHY FAMILY

"The natural healing force within each of us is the greatest force in getting well."

—HIPPOCRATES

ONCE I LEARNED enough from my community to feel like I could talk to my family and others confidently about the subject (I am still learning), and once I lived through enough experiences and learned what works and what does not—for my family, anyway—I began to compile these steps. You may add to them, or you may have done some of these already—either way, check through this list and try these steps with your family. The most important factors are for you to be determined to get well, to have faith that you will, and to be UNSTOPPABLE in trying new things until you discover what works.

Six Steps to a Healthy Family

1. Eliminate exposure to all harmful chemicals, antibiotics, and GMOs.

This means avoid all conventional food and eat only organic as much as possible, because the majority of the conventional food in our country is contaminated.

Discontinue the use of mainstream popular bath and body care products, as well as household cleaners. Use only nontoxic products (read the ingredients) or cleaners for the home like vinegar, baking soda, and essential oils.

Avoid antibiotics. Many antibiotics have been reported to cause tears in tendons and other severe reactions. Some people build antibiotic resistance. One dose of antibiotics can disrupt gut flora for two years.

Install a reverse osmosis water filter or good filter tested to remove heavy metals, pesticides, and glyphosate specifically. (Glyphosate is different from other pesticides.) If you do use reverse osmosis, be sure to clean the filter yearly and add trace minerals back into the water, as they have been removed. I do not recommend buying bottled water unless your tap water is truly toxic, as most bottled water is just tap water anyway and by buying it you contribute to plastic in landfills.

2. Detox.

Either test your family for glyphosate, heavy metals, and other toxins *or* simply assume your family has ingested toxins (which is a safe assumption in America today) and begin a detox plan. Labs such as Health Research Institute, Microbe Inotech, The Detox Project, or Great Plains Labs have glyphosate or toxin tests ranging from $100–400 per test.

There are many detox plans, including Chinese herbal, homeopathic, psyllium husk drinks, activated charcoal, eating cilantro or herbs such as dandelion, burdock, milk thistle, cellular detoxes, chelation therapy, and benzonite clay, to name a few. The most effective detox is sweating. This is free and healthy for you. If you cannot afford a sauna or membership to a gym with a sauna, you can get a tracksuit and run or exercise for free.

You may also get genetic testing to see if you/your family has the methylenetetrahydrofolate reductase (MTHFR) gene mutation (about 20 percent or more of the population is estimated to have this), which means a possible inability to detox chemicals properly. This can help with determining with a medical professional the direction, length of time, and type of detox that is needed. Or, if you cannot afford the tests, you can simply assume your body needs help detoxing and just take steps like the above to detox.

Keep in mind that when the body is detoxing, the imbalance of pathogenic bacteria in the gut that is likely the source of all the inflammation, rashes, and behavioral or learning issues. These issues tend to recede as the bad bacteria get balanced from all the goodness your child or family member is putting in his/her gut. That bad bacteria dying off will make things look like they are getting worse before they get better. So after about a week or so, expect the rashes to get worse, behavioral issues to act up, and for your child to have pretty demanding cravings. Children with an overgrowth of bad gut bacteria will fiercely crave dairy, wheat, and sweets. Don't give in and give up on healing! Do yourself a favor and do not have those items in the house! Have lots of healthy, fresh, organic fruits that your kids can grab on their own, and your life will be so much easier.

3. Restore your gut.

If you can, get your child or family member tested for fungus, pathogenic gut bacteria, and the state of their gut biome. Eliminating the toxins and antibiotics helps to reduce inflammation and continued damage to the gut lining but will not repair the damage as quickly as introducing supportive supplements. Restore for Gut Health, GI Revive, MSM by MRM, and Colloidal Silver are just a few that are reported to either zipper together the tight junctions of the stomach or coat the stomach to support cell repair. Natural antibiotics and natural antifungals like goldenseal tincture and plantain tea are much easier on the body, affordable, and can be just as effective as over-the-counter antibiotics.

If you have extensive gut dysbiosis and health issues you may want to look into food sensitivities to lectins (grains, peanuts, soy, and seafood), nightshades (eggplants, tomatoes, peppers, and potatoes) and the FODMAPS (an acronym for foods that are known for triggering the symptoms of digestive problems—fermentable oligo-, di-, monosaccharides and polyols) or GAPS (Gut and Psychology Syndrome) diet. Repair of the gut cannot begin if you are still exposing the gut to offending foods.

4. Reduce inflammation.

Avoiding pesticides like glyphosate and foods with lectins (beans, nightshades, wheat, and even fermented food for some), which can cause inflammation in some people, is just as important as avoiding GMOs. Once you have eliminated the source of the inflammation, a supplement to try is Elite Active H2. This molecular hydrogen water tablet supplement turns free radicals mostly made up of oxygen and hydrogen (OH) molecules, into water. The OH in our bodies grabs on to one of the H molecular hydrogen molecules (made up of two hydrogen (HH) molecules) from the supplement, and becomes H20. So free radicals, which are a major source of inflammation, can be turned into innocuous water. Hemp oil, such as Colorado Hemp Oil, can also reduce the signals to the autoimmune microglial cells that trigger inflammation. Both are available on Momsacrossamerica.org as fundraisers for our programs.

5. Balance gut bacteria.

Unlike any other time in history, due to the toxins in our environment and food, American moms, caregivers, and all people around the world must turn their attention to gut flora (also called gut microbiome, or gut bacteria), which harbors 70 percent of the immune system. Studies show that probiotics improve "good" gut bacteria and reduce autism symptoms in rats. Mothers of children with autism have had the same experience. Probiotics are one step in restoring gut health by restoring the balance of "good" bacteria and "bad" bacteria.

Dr. Zach Bush, a triple board-certified MD, says, "I think we are going to find that there really are no 'good' or 'bad' bacteria—they each play a role." For instance, the Bacteroides fragilis bacteria, which has been shown to reverse autism-like behavior in mice, is also a pathogen and can cause infections, so it is not available for purchase. What this means is that we just have to make sure we have a balance of bacteria—not an overgrowth of "bad" bacteria like E. coli and salmonella, which is what is happening in the majority of children today. The best way to balance the gut is through food: fermented foods such as organic yogurt, kefir, sauerkraut, and fermented vegetables can put up to a trillion good bacteria in the gut in a serving.

Some children have such extensive gut damage that probiotics are necessary for a short term. Mothers report that their children begin to sleep better or focus on tasks more efficiently after the introduction of a probiotic. Probiotic supplements are beneficial to reintroduce bacteria that may have been killed off by glyphosate or prescribed antibiotics but are not optimal for long-term reliability to balance the gut flora. The reason is that most probiotic supplements only contain six to ten different strains of bacteria. Our body is supposed to have thirty thousand different strains. So, thinking that taking a supplement with just ten strains of probiotics is going to balance out the gut bacteria, without changing your diet, is misunderstanding the gut biome. Most people, including doctors, don't know this, so don't feel badly if you didn't! If you do take probiotics, make sure to also take prebiotics—and also make sure they are high quality and organic.

6. Replenish minerals.

Because of chemical farming and industrial pollutants, which kill off good bacteria and soil microbes, the soil our food—even organic food—is grown in is massively nutrient deficient. I asked Dr. Don Huber to look at nutritional content tests I was given on carrots and tomatoes by an owner of a fertilizer company and he said, "If they came from my farm I would be embarrassed to call that food. The mineral content is almost nonexistent—especially the zinc." Many minerals are being depleted from food by chemical farming. If you wanted to get the same amount of iron from spinach today as from a serving of spinach from the 1950s, you would have to eat seventy-five servings. Eating a whole, organic, local, seasonal, plant-based diet is an important step to take to restore minerals, but it may not be enough if you have health issues and deficiencies. Get your child or family tested for mineral deficiencies. Some children with autism, or elderly people with dementia, may need methyl B-12 shots—not just supplements—as the children's and senior's absorption capabilities may be dysfunctional. It would be safe to assume that we are all deficient in trace minerals as well, considering the chelating function of glyphosate, and taking a trace mineral supplement is highly effective and easy. Moms Across America has sourced trace minerals, and a list of foods rich in them, that taste good, and are of high quality can be found on our website under health solutions.

If your child has autism, I suggest you research what many report having great success with: biomedical intervention, CBD oil, chelation therapy, eating organic food, eliminating gluten and dairy, methyl B-12 shots, and natural antifungals and antibiotics. Others report that the GAPS (Gut and Psychology Syndrome) diet, Body Ecology Diet, or Elimination Diet worked wonders for their gut issues. The point is to keep trying. Do not give up. You can recover your child's health.

How I Helped My Child to Eat Healthy Foods

Once you have the information about GMOs, how do you help your kids to switch to healthy foods?

"When you know better, you do better," said Maya Angelou. This means that each person should know for themselves. Imposing what you know on others does not mean they will do better. For most people, having their children become aware of how they feel when they eat certain foods and take ownership of their own health, is the best way. Once *they* know for themselves, they do better.

After years of struggling with milk, nut, food dye, wheat/gluten, and many more allergies my son and I were both exhausted. One day, when Ben was about nine years old, he sat forlornly at the breakfast counter with a rash around his mouth and said, "I wish all my allergies would go away."

Without his saying more, we both thought about how awful his new, mysterious allergy had been over the past seven months—a painful, red rash around his mouth and swollen, flaking lips that lasted for weeks at a time. The rash would eventually go away but then a few weeks later it would come back, and we had no idea why. It was embarrassing and frustrating for both of us. He was tired. I was, too. My heart hurt for him. We had both had enough.

I said sadly, "Yeah. Me, too, buddy," but I thought, *That will never happen—we just have to live with it.* Then I realized I was being resigned and doubtful about my abilities. I was being disempowered. I was also seeing *him* as small, as someone who could not do anything about his own health. Suddenly, that did not work for me.

I began to wonder—what if his allergies could go away? I thought of our cousin Sara in San Francisco who had recently told us that she ate gluten-free for a year and after that she could now eat gluten now and then and not be severely affected.

So I reminded my son about Sara and then I asked, "Ben, what if you could eat pizza now and then at a party a year from now? Not all the time, but once in a while. Would you like that?" Suddenly, he knew he could do better.

His eyes lit up, he sat up straight, and he said emphatically, *"Yes!"*

I realized I could choose to see his allergies as an opportunity. So, I did.

"Ben, would you be my partner in your health? Will you do *whatever it takes*? Drink green drinks? Go to alternative doctors? Eat organic?" I felt alive with excitement.

He nodded and again said, "Yes!" He chose to take on his own health.

"Okay. It's a deal, "I said, and we shook hands.

We had created a partnership!

I then looked him in the eye, while still holding his hand, and with all my heart I said, "Ben, I promise you that you will get better." I got chills when I said it. I made that promise even when I did not know how I would do it, because I knew making that happen would require both of us to take new actions we might never normally take. He would have to have faith and take strength in our partnership. I would be compelled by my promise—my word—to find a way. My integrity was on the line, and that was a big deal.

When his allergies cleared up a few months later, and he had only a barely perceptible reaction, I celebrated him. I high fived him, looked him in the eye and said," You did this! *You* are healing yourself. You are making awesome choices and your body can process the allergens now! You are getting better! Woohoo!" I did a happy dance until it was almost embarrassing.

The funny thing was that when a year later came, he didn't want to eat conventional pizza at birthday parties. Now, he doesn't even want to walk into McDonald's to use the bathroom. He chooses to eat only organic foods, and his good choices give me peace of mind that is better than any other reward I could imagine.

Five Steps to Have Your Child Eat Healthy Foods

1. Be ready for change.
Both you and your family member—say, your son—must be at a place in your lives where you can acknowledge that the current situation is not working. You both must be ready to make changes.

If you think he might not be aware that it is time to make changes, simply ask him about how he feels about where he is right now. How do you feel when you eat XYZ food? Do you feel good? Bad? Do you want to keep feeling that way? What happens when you feel bad? Are you grumpy? Do you get in fights with your sister and lose TV time? Do you get time-outs? Help him answer these questions until he realizes how much his body is impacted and sees that it is time to make changes.

2. Help him imagine the possibilities.
Ask him: What else could be possible? Wonder what if . . . you could eat bread or a slice of pizza (or whatever his favorite food is) a year from now and be okay? Let your son describe what that would be like. Let him imagine himself feeling good and eating the food he loves.

3. Ask for partnership.
Ask your child to be your partner in health. Will he or she learn new things, work with you, drink green drinks, and eat organic foods? You will be his or her partner. He or she will not be alone.

You will benefit from a partner, too—another mom, parent, spouse, or health coach. Your buddy would ideally do a weekly or daily call with you to support and hold each other accountable for what you are up to with your dietary changes. It does not have to be a strictly structured setup. To be most effective you would ask that person if she could be your accountability buddy. Your goal could include getting your family healthy (including yourself). This person will be a sounding board and support. Discuss whether she would agree to speak on a certain day or a certain number of times a week. Don't assume. When you talk with your buddy, make sure not only to allow yourself space to complain about how hard it is, but to share solutions and acknowledge each other for your accomplishments. Most importantly, listen to her, too. Her struggles with getting healthy can be your greatest lessons. Do this regularly, without fail. The more accountability you put yourself on the hook for, the more results you will produce. Plus, when you have support, you can better support your son or family.

4. Make a promise to your child that his or her health will improve.
You may not know how this will happen when you make the promise, but you will both take actions that you otherwise would not have taken. When you draw a line in the sand, you step up.

A promise changes the actions a person takes, and this alters the results. Without a promise, we usually don't take action. Actions such as putting reverse osmosis (RO) on your kitchen tap, adding sauerkraut, organic yogurt, and miso to your diet, and taking daily supplements such as the ones we offer as solutions on our website. With a promise we take new actions and then we show up.

5. Celebrate any and all wins.
Be sure to celebrate all victories with delight, a reward, and quality time together. Focus on the improvements and acknowledge what you have learned from any setbacks. Your son's health might seem like it's in the toilet, but when he has gone a week having a big green salad every day for the first time in his life, celebrating it with a special fishing trip or going to the dollar theater to watch a funny movie, just the two of you, makes everything right in the world.

Finally, remember that every day brings a choice. Do not berate him if he whines or complains. Instead, acknowledge that it is not easy, but remind him of his choice—his commitment to partnership and to make himself better. Tell him you have faith in him—he can do it. Do not allow any anger to come into the conversation, just understanding and support. Always make it about him, not you, and he will see that he himself is in charge of his health. The good choices you support him in making now, while he is under your roof, will go with him, and empower him, when he is a young man, healthy and responsible, making a difference for others out in the world.

When I learned about GMOs, my primary concern was my own family, and whether or not my children would choose to eat non-GMO and organic on their own someday. At first, I wasn't ready to focus on other people as well. But when my nine-year-old son Ben thought about his classmates and asked if he could give a presentation on the subject, it was a turning point for me. I didn't have to worry about him and his choices—he was fine . . . and already focusing on helping others. He realized "the kids that were making the teacher yell all day were the ones eating GMO junk food." His thinking was that if they don't eat GMO food, maybe the teacher wouldn't yell so much. On the third day of school, he stood up in front of his new combo fourth/fifth-grade class and proudly gave his presentation called "Healthy, Happy Students." Later, he won a citizenship award. Parents told me that their children were very impressed by his presentation and stopped eating Cheetos and other GMO foods. Ben's courage to speak up in front of his class inspired me to declare that I, too, would be a public speaker on the subject. Within a few months, I was being asked to speak at expos and went on to be sponsored to speak internationally, in countries I had always dreamed of visiting.

A few months after Ben's talk, with the support of many generous people, I started Moms Across America (MAA), a national coalition of UNSTOPPABLE moms. I was thrilled to have a nonprofit fiscal sponsor, who was then called the California State Grange (now the California Guild), led by Bob McFarland. Our motto is "Empowered Moms, Healthy Kids." Our mission is: *To empower millions to educate themselves about GMOs and related toxins, offer GMO-free and organic solutions, and support local leadership to create healthy communities.* As we connected with thousands of people each day through social media and our website, I began hearing from other mothers that their children were getting better by avoiding GMOs and eating organic. It felt like we were on a surging tidal wave of mothers rising up to protect our families, and it was thrilling.

Shopping for Healthy Food

Unlike our grandmothers, who could shop without paying much regard to the labels on their food and could easily identify what the ingredients were, we have a very different landscape in the grocery store.

Today we can buy meals in a box with fifty unpronounceable mystery ingredients. These meals will feed our whole family if we simply heat the plastic package for a few minutes in a microwave (leaching estrogenic hormones from the plastic while we're at it) or thirty minutes in the oven (during which that time you could have cooked a fresh meal, by the way). But it's challenging to resist the apparent convenience. I call it the "disease of ease" when the choices for convenience overtake us. We can become too accustomed to fast, cheap, tasty, and easy. We too often grab the cheap, processed, GMO, packaged snacks and frozen dinners because they are convenient. It's not worth it, however, when you understand the impact on your family's health.

To start eliminating GMOs and toxins from your food and water, you will first want to know what all the labels on the packages mean. There are many different labels on food products these days, however, so I will address the differences.

Natural (Baloney)

"Natural," "made with natural ingredients," and "100 percent natural" mean nothing. The word looks appealing and you may feel slightly better reaching for the granola bars made with 100 percent natural oats, but you would unfortunately be mistaken. None of these claims mean that the product does not contain genetically modified ingredients or pesticides. This fact is very disturbing, but absolutely true. Many kinds of so-called natural products have been tested and have been found to contain GMOs and pesticides. This is because the FDA does not require "natural" to mean only truly natural ingredients—no GMOs or pesticides. At the time of writing this book, the FDA does not have a definition of "natural," and is only now considering, after several lawsuits over the issue have been brought against food manufacturers, defining the term.

Moms Across America, Organic Consumers Association, and Beyond Pesticides, with the Richman Law Group, sued Nature Valley over the presence of glyphosate in their oatmeal bars. Whether the courts find this acceptable or not is yet to be seen. Either way, more and more consumers find this unacceptable every day, and will not buy products even if their labels say that they are "natural."

Non-GMO Project Verified (Not Good Enough)
Many people now buy products that are labeled "Non-GMO Project Verified" and feel that they are buying a safer product for their families. This is also not the case. Non-GMO Project Verified only means it was tested and contains less than 0.9 percent GMOs. This is a good thing—however, it does NOT mean that the product does not contain toxic pesticides. The label has gained a huge amount of ground in the marketplace. Many companies have spent thousands of dollars per product to obtain that verification, and most consumers now know what GMOs are, partially due to this label. Although I am grateful that the Non-GMO Project Verified team efforts have raised awareness about GMOs, many customers are now confused and value the Non-GMO Project Verified label over the USDA organic label. This is a dangerous misunderstanding. People consuming Non-GMO Project Verified foods are very often still exposing themselves to toxic pesticides. People who eat organic, for the most part (drift contamination happens in small amounts, and some mislabeling has been recorded), are not.

Organic (GMO-Free and More!)
Organic, on the other hand, means that the food ingredients are not GMO, and toxic herbicides are not permitted in growing them. The pesticides used have been approved by the National Organic Standards Board (NOSB) and are predominately natural. There are different levels of organic. To be 100 percent organic, it must be 100 percent. USDA Organic means 95 percent organic. "Made with organic ingredients" means it must contain 70 percent organic ingredients. This also means the other 30 percent could be GMO and/or contaminated with toxic chemicals. The problem is that the organic certification program, run by the USDA, does not perform consistent GMO or pesticide testing to confirm that contamination has not occurred. They do test, but not consistently. So, contamination can and does occur—usually in small amounts. This is why knowing your farmer and eating locally grown food is the best option.

Buying items like pasta, cereal, or crackers that are 100 percent organic or that have the USDA organic label *and* the Non-GMO Project Verified label is preferred. Even better, if available, are products labeled "biodynamic." Biodynamic means that not only do the growers not use GMOs and toxic chemicals as the organic label requires, but they tend to the soil, grow beneficial plants to add minerals to the soil, and improve the quality of the crops by working with nature. Biodynamic foods tend to have much higher nutritional content than conventional and organic foods.

One should note fair trade certified does not mean 100 percent organic. It

SOME SYMBOLS TO LOOK FOR:

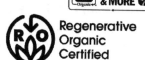

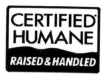

is reported by fairtradecertifed.org that only about 50 percent of their certified products are organic. Grass-fed also does not mean organic. According to the American Grassfed Association, they do allow for farmers to spray their hay and alfalfa crops with glyphosate before harvest. It is not a common practice, but it is not disallowed and does happen in northern, wetter regions. Glyphosate free, certified locally owned, and certified humane, all important certifications, also do not mean organic.

If you cannot afford to buy 100 percent organic, at least switch your baked goods and grain products to organic to reduce your exposure to glyphosate. To avoid the most common GMO foods, cut out corn, soy, and processed foods. Eating whole, local, seasonal foods is the best way to stay healthy.

Food Allergies

An important reason why most people read labels these days is the rise of food allergies. Common allergens now include wheat, milk, soy, corn, peanuts, nuts, food dyes, and eggs. If you think about it, these ingredients are in most of the prepared foods on the shelf, making grocery shopping more of a minefield experience than ever before. It was not like this when I was a child. Food allergies in children have increased 400 percent since GMOs and glyphosate were introduced into our food supply. Over 150 children have been reported to die each year from food allergies, and millions more experience life-threatening or serious reactions. I believe that this is a result of what has been done to the food—it is not the fault of our children's bodies or the actual food itself. Adults are also affected. I was recently bicycling through an Oregon neighborhood wearing my "GMO, We're Not Buying It!" T-shirt when a man in his sixties shouted to me, "I am trying to read your shirt!"

I called back, "It says, GMO, We're Not Buying It! Do you know about GMOs?"

He replied, "Yes I do! They are the reason for my allergies! I can't go to a restaurant without an EpiPen because I might go into anaphylactic shock! I know all about GMOs!"

The problem with ingredient labeling is that many ingredients are not clearly identified. Ingredients such as soy lecithin are obviously made from soy—however, one would never expect that monosodium glutamate, gelatin, carob, autolyzed yeast, oyster sauce, fish sauce, texturized vegetable protein, vegetable broth, vegetable starch, or natural flavoring would contain soy. Over 90 percent of the soy crops in the United States are GMO.

Corn (which is predominantly GMO) is also hiding out in many food products. Citric acid, confectioner's sugar, dextrin, dextrose, fructose, lactic acid, monosodium glutamate, sorbitol, and starch can all contain corn—just to name a few.

Getting both you and your family tested and finding out what you are all allergic to is crucial for good health these days. Most people tested find out they are allergic to things that they commonly eat and had no idea could be affecting them. Too many of us think that feeling tired, irritable, or forgetful is normal. Finding out what foods you are allergic to and taking steps to avoid them can change your life and the lives of the people around you. For many children, who are the most susceptible, avoiding allergens can be lifesaving.

How to Avoid Food Allergy Attacks

- Read every label. Always. Never assume a different flavor of the same brand of cookie/food will be nut-free/allergen-free just because the one you normally buy is.

- Do not serve your child anything at a potluck that you didn't make or that is not a whole food such as an apple. For example, avoid salads, guacamole, or home baked muffins—they all could have nuts.

- If you do serve your child someone else's dish, only do so if you have spoken to the person who made the food and asked them specifically about the ingredients your child is allergic to when this person is not tired, rushed, or drunk.

- Make sure utensils that have come in contact with allergens are not used to serve food to your child.

- Advise all caretakers in person and in writing of your child's allergies.

- Always carry snacks with you and bring your own food to parties. I tell my family, "We are going to this birthday party to celebrate Joshua, not the food. We have our own tasty, organic snacks."

- *Always* carry an EpiPen (or a similar, less expensive epinephrine brand) and Benadryl and give a second set to all caretakers.

- If your child does eat an allergen and is just experiencing a mild rash, have them immediately drink two glasses of water to flush out food more quickly. If they can vomit the food out of their body, that may help alleviate the reaction.

- If any swelling occurs anywhere on the body go immediately to the ER after administering the epinephrine.

- If you cannot afford the allergy tests your doctor recommends and are experiencing allergy symptoms, you may want to try what is called the elimination diet. Eliminate the most common allergy foods for two weeks to a month and see how you feel. Reintroduce them into your diet, see how you feel, and adjust your diet accordingly. Many people have resolved their health issues by taking these simple steps.

Gluten-Free

Millions of Americans now also seek out the label "gluten-free" or "GF." In 2014, statistics showed that one out of four women over the age of thirty had a gluten intolerance, and most were unaware of it. Symptoms of a gluten intolerance can include bloating, weight gain, rashes, bumps on the upper arms, fatigue, headaches, brain fog, and irritability. People with a gluten intolerance can be extremely edgy, quick to anger, and have a hard time controlling themselves. I know this from firsthand experience, and so does my husband. I am convinced that gluten intolerance is the unidentified reason for many divorces, and I am grateful to my husband for his patience. For people trying to regain energy and lose weight, going completely gluten-free—not just partially gluten-free—is crucial. Gluten can remain in the body for months.

Gluten-free foods are important for people with a gluten intolerance, full-on gluten allergy, or Celiac disease. Most gluten-free foods however, are *not* also organic. So once again, people often think they are eating more healthy food, when in fact they could also be eating toxic chemicals.

It is important for gluten-free foods to be both gluten-free and organic. If you cannot find gluten-free *and* organic bread, baked goods, or pasta, it may be possible to eat organic ancient grain products. This is explained by Cyndi O'Meara, producer and director of the documentary *What's With Wheat?* Modern wheat has been modified to contain a new protein called gliadin. Dr. William Davis explains in his blog "Wheat Belly" that the gliadin protein of wheat degrades in the gastrointestinal tract to small polypeptides that act as opiates called exorphins—causing addictive eating, food obsession, and incessant hunger. Removal of the gliadin generates a withdrawal syndrome. (Which can mean aggravated behavior.)

Many people, like myself, who are intolerant to wheat or gluten only test positive for an intolerance to the gliadin protein and none of the other proteins. This means that I can eat ancient grains with no issues. These ancient grains, however, should also be organic.

Many people who react to wheat and gluten products may be reacting simply because of the glyphosate sprayed on the wheat crops as a drying agent. One can see and feel the difference when traveling to countries such as Germany, France, or Italy where the practice of desiccating wheat and other crops with glyphosate has been discontinued. I recently went to Switzerland and France and could eat bread for breakfast, lunch, and dinner and did not once get a rash, fatigue, or irritability. Going gluten-free makes a huge difference for many people, but going organic should be the first thing that people with reactions to wheat should try. Below are some things to consider when shopping for gluten-free and healthy food in order to save money.

Saving Money, Eating Healthy

The most important part of feeding your family healthy food is to get the unhealthy foods out of the house entirely. If you don't buy it, your kids can't eat it! (Not at your house anyway!)

Produce

A plant-based diet can save you a lot of money, reduce health issues, costs, and be very satisfying. Growing your own vegetables is the best way to know whether or not they have been sprayed with chemicals. Supporting your local farmer's market is great for the local economy, as the farmers make many times more profit selling directly to the consumer than through a supermarket. If you do buy produce from a grocery store, buying frozen organic vegetables in bulk can save money and also reduce food waste.

Bread and Other Baked Goods

Read the labels carefully. If you cannot find both gluten-free and organic, gluten-free breads that do not contain soy, corn, canola, or sugar (the biggest offenders of GMOs and glyphosate) are safer. If you are gluten intolerant but do not have Celiac disease, you may be able to tolerate bread made from an organic ancient grain such as kamut, spelt, or einkorn grains. Avoid conventional whole wheat bread. Contrary to the current understanding that whole wheat is better than white bread, recent testing shows that whole wheat has a much higher level of glyphosate than white bread. This is because the shells of the wheat kernels are left on and have been sprayed with glyphosate.

The most cost-efficient bread is homemade, costing about one dollar per loaf instead of four to five dollars for organic, store-bought bread. Many online grocery stores or co-ops like Azure Standard sell bulk organic sprouted rice grain flour, ancient grains, organic tapioca, potato starch, and sorghum flour. It helps to get a bread machine that also works for making pizza dough. Make more than one batch of pizza dough at a time and freeze the unused portion. Previously prepared organic pizza dough can be a lifesaver on a night with sports and homework looming ahead.

Buying five- or twenty-five-pound sacks of flour and mixing your own baking mix saves you about four dollars per meal of pancakes for a family of five. It's worth it. I use the baking mix recipe from the book *15 Minute Healthy, Organic Meals for Less than $10 a Day* by Susan Patterson. I mix eight cups of baking mix at a time in a brown paper shopping bag, shake it up, and store it in a glass, airtight canister. When you first get organic flour, you need to freeze it for 3 days before storing it in the pantry as sometimes moths can be present, particularly because pest-killing chemicals are not used at any stage in the flour, and freezing kills them. Always store flours, beans, and pasta in airtight containers, whether organic or not.

Crackers

Avoid conventional whole grain crackers due to likely high glyphosate residues. Organic and gluten-free crackers are available in most grocery stores, and definitely online. An added benefit to gluten-free and organic crackers is that some brands include flaxseeds and other ingredients that are far more nutritious than highly processed wheat flour.

Pasta

The type of pasta that you buy is important. Quinoa can have glyphosate levels of up to 5 ppm unless it is organic. Corn can have up to 13 ppm of glyphosate in America. Rice may also have some glyphosate residues. Buckwheat has tested high in glyphosate, so avoid buckwheat noodles unless they are organic. Whether the pasta is gluten-free or not, it must be organic grain for you to avoid glyphosate. Alternatives to grain pasta are curly cut zucchini or spaghetti squash, which both make very hearty "noodles."

Meat

If my family buys meat—which is very rare now that my eldest son has gone vegan—we alternate between buying from a farmer we know, local ranches' grass-fed beef at a farmer's market, and grocery store organic meat. Grass-fed meat is generally considered better because, if the animals are *entirely* grass-fed (and not grain finished—meaning fed grains during the last few months to "fatten them up"), the animals have not been fed GMO grain sprayed with glyphosate. However, grass-fed does not necessarily mean glyphosate-free grass. In wetter northern regions, some hay farmers might spray their crops with glyphosate as a drying agent, so it's best to know your farmer and his or her practices. Although organically raised meat products are more expensive, the taste and quality are superior and well worth the higher cost. Buying a bulk "share" of a cow or pig can reduce the cost of fine cuts of meat by 50 percent. Ask a nearby ranch for a share and get your neighbors to chip in.

My family buys frozen fish when we can find wild caught, never farmed fish, to avoid antibiotics and toxins. More and more often now we chose meat alternatives or just eat lots of vegetables. I have been pleasantly surprised that a large curry stir-fry leaves me completely satisfied and not craving meat at all. In addition, I feel good that my choice can improve my health as well as prevent pollution in our environment.

According to cardiologist Dr. Joel Kahn and many studies, reducing red meat consumption is very important for lowering the risk of heart disease and cancer. In addition, concentrated animal feeding operations (CAFOs) impact climate change. The methane that factory farmed, GMO fed cows emit is just as damaging to the environment as fossil fuels. GMO crops grown to feed the cows use toxins that deplete the soil and reduce its ability to absorb carbon, which many scientists believe is the leading reason for climate change. The runoff from factory farms is linked to the dead zones in the oceans. The high capacity wells needed to supply the feedlots are also impacting local residents who rely on that same water supply. Twenty-five hundred gallons of water are required to produce the feed to yield one pound of beef. Eating vegetarian or vegan as much as possible is often better for you, the environment, and all of us. It is also much less expensive. Just make sure you buy organic, as vegan and vegetarian crop ingredients can also be heavily sprayed with glyphosate.

Sauces

Organic gluten-free enzymes taste just like soy sauce. There are several organic and gluten-free mustards, ketchups, and barbecue sauce brands available today. Most of these are also healthier than nonorganic sauces because they do not contain high fructose corn syrup. Keep in mind that many sauces (as well as lunch meats, milks, ice cream, and other creamy foods) contain carrageenan, a highly processed food filler that has been shown to lead to stomach ulcers and could lead to cancer. The National Organic Standards Board disallowed carrageenan in organic food in 2016, but the USDA, likely pressured by big food corporations, overruled their decision and allowed carrageenan in organic foods in 2018. Much more work needs to be done to have carrageenan banned altogether . . . and to get money out of politics.

Soups, Beans, and Potatoes

Keep in mind that nonorganic rye and barley contain gluten and can also have high glyphosate residues, so watch out for them in soups. Organic gluten-free broth is readily available in the stores but if I buy meat, I buy organic chickens (air dried is best to avoid chemical wash) and use the leftovers to make broth and a Chinese chicken porridge called jook with rice, ginger, gluten-free soy sauce, and chicken. Hearty and delicious!

Buying bulk organic lentils or beans and making soup in a slow cooker yields twelve servings for the same price as one can of beans. Add a grass-fed beef bone for a meatier flavor or curry for a tasty vegan meal.

Do you love French fries? You can save $917 in a year for a family of five just from making and eating French fries at home two times a week instead of in a restaurant. A meal of dressed up baked potatoes and salad for a whole family can cost less than one meal out at a restaurant.

Oatmeal

Oatmeal is generally considered a very healthy way to start the day and is often one of the first foods given to babies. The fact is that, unless it is organic, it is allowed to contain high levels of glyphosate. Oat products *must* be organic *and* "certified gluten-free" (which means the product has been tested to be sure it has less than 20 ppm of gluten) in order to avoid gluten. Otherwise, the oats could have been cross-contaminated with wheat, barley, and/or rye during the handling and processing of the oats. Gluten-free but nonorganic means it has likely been sprayed with glyphosate as a drying agent.

Buying organic oats in bulk is far less expensive than buying smaller amounts and is a great way to save money on expensive snack foods. You can make three dozen oatmeal bars on Sunday for snacks for the week ahead for two to three dollars, rather than spending five to six dollars on one box containing six organic granola bars or three to four dollars for conventional. When people say organic is "too expensive," they usually are not considering buying in bulk and cooking at home. The fact is that eating organic at home is far cheaper than the standard American diet when you eat out, and far cheaper than doctors' bills, too.

> *I choose to eat organic food whenever possible because I believe it's better for my health, the environment, and the farmers who grow our food. Organic crops aren't grown with synthetic pesticides like Roundup herbicide, which is polluting our water, land, air, and bodies. Some people don't realize that non-GMO crops can be sprayed with Roundup, too, in addition to all the other chemicals used on conventional crops. There are non-GMO products on the market that seem "healthy," but are still laced with Roundup and other synthetic pesticides—and that's just one reason why organic is a healthier choice. Buying quality organic food and eating the most nutritious foods on the planet can save you big bucks down the road in medical costs, prescription drugs, and visits to the doctor—it's totally up to you to make it a priority.*
>
> —Vani Hari, New York Times bestselling author and founder of FoodBabe.com

Changing your diet may seem extremely drastic at first, and you may be so unsure about what to eat that you may not eat as often as before. Not eating as often can leave you cranky and more likely to "cheat" and eat unhealthy foods. Don't do this to yourself and your family. Make sure that you and the kids eat some form of protein every two hours such as organic nuts, yogurt, oatmeal bars, beans, or raw veggies (yes, vegetables contain protein!) because you are not getting heavily processed food that sits in your stomach for four hours. Eating this way is healthier and closer to the way we are meant to eat.

> The ticket to triumph in health issues comes when you value yourself and your family's health more than you do convenience. When you see abstaining from harmful foods as a gift to your family, rather than a deprivation, and choose healthy, whole, organic foods, you can shift their health, happiness, and future in a matter of weeks. You are all worth it.

Eating organic at home can be less expensive than the standard American diet eaten out and is often faster than driving to a restaurant and waiting for service.

Susan Patterson, author of *15 Minute Healthy, Organic Meals for Less Than $10 a Day*, shares:

> While I wanted to make sure my children were fed right, as a single, widowed, full-time working mom, I had to figure out how to do that on a budget in a way that took no time as I didn't have any. I experimented and experimented and found out that organic rice and beans only costs thirty cents more a pound than nonorganic, so I made that my mainstay. In order to save time when I was cooking one meal, as long as I was in the kitchen, I put together ingredients for a second or third meal. For instance, while I was barbecuing Sunday dinner, I would put on some rice to cook in a rice cooker and beans in a Crock-Pot, so I didn't need to watch them and then added some marinated chicken to the grill. It doesn't take any longer to grill meat for a second meal. Then during the week, my children can take the rice, beans, and chicken and add some frozen corn to a double boiler top. In five minutes, it is all steamed up. Then they just add some avocado, hot sauce, etc. for a bowl or burrito that cost me three dollars. Believe me, three dollars to feed a teenager is a bargain. This way I didn't get text after text beginning at four o'clock, "I'm starving, when are you going to be home?"
>
> On Sunday, in twenty to thirty minutes I could easily prepare four meals ahead of time. With practice and persistence, I know anyone can make it work to eat organic!

Dining Out As Safely As Possible

If you are eating out at a restaurant, always search first for organic and, if you need to, gluten-free options, which are more likely to be found in mom and pop cafes versus chain restaurants. We often ask the restaurant if they have organic options—and if they don't, we leave. If, for instance, you are traveling and organic absolutely cannot be found, the best food to eat is Indian curry because they usually do not use canola oil (typically GMO) in the sauces and are traditionally rice or potato based making them gluten-free.

Chinese dishes without MSG and breaded meat, like steamed or grilled meat are better than tofu, which is usually made of GMO soy. Just skip the brown sauces.

Mexican bowls of rice and beans are a better option than flour tortillas—and skip the corn kernels or corn tortillas. (Over 90 percent of corn in Mexico was recently found to contain GMOs.) If you really want to eat the chips and salsa, always go for the blue corn, which is not GMO.

Japanese sushi or dishes are a decent dining out option, except for the breaded or tempura items. Avoid the miso soup and soy sauce (not gluten free), which are likely GMO soy.

American food is unfortunately the least desirable option, especially fried food, because wheat is added as a filler or coating to almost everything and is likely highly contaminated with glyphosate. In addition, most American food is cooked in canola, cottonseed, or corn oil, which is all GMO and can have up to 40 ppm of glyphosate.

I love my country but going out to eat at an American diner and having a GMO sandwich, burgers, or fish and chips is no longer an option for our family. GMO companies like Monsanto have ruined the pleasure of dining out for us unless we can find an organic restaurant. Fortunately, more and more restaurants are figuring out that customers want organic and are making the switch. Chef Patrick Stark of Sundown at Granada in Texas shared with me that his sales have increased by $10,000 a week, compared to the previous years' sales, since he went primarily GMO-free and organic. Encourage your favorite local restaurant to go organic and you could create a win-win for everyone!

CHAPTER SIX
TOXINS IN DAILY LIFE

"Change is the end result of all true learning."
—LEO BUSCAGLIA

ALLERGIES DO NOT begin and end in the kitchen. We never thought about my son Ben's carrageenan allergy when we took him to the dentist until he broke out in a rash. Who could have imagined that an allergen would be found in toothpaste? I thought I had enough to worry about with fluoride—which has been proven to be a neurotoxin—and yet, fluoride is added to toothpaste and cavity treatments. Now we know carrageenan is in most toothpastes which can be dangerous too! Parents never used to ask what was in the toothpaste a dentist used—we just trusted that it was safe. The fact is that, as exhausting as it can be, we now must question everything.

Over the counter medications, toothpaste, suntan lotions, clothing detergents, fabric softeners, and body care products are more likely to give a child a contact reaction today than they were in years past. More chemicals are being allowed in our products than ever before. Toxins from nonstick pans, flame retardant on pajamas and sofas, formaldehyde in many kitchen cabinets, off-gassing from rubber turf playgrounds, aerial spraying, plastic food packaging, car exhaust and jet fuel, toxins in our drinking water and medications are all inundating our children. In fact, over eighty thousand chemicals have been approved by the EPA since the 1940s and hundreds of those are endocrine disruptors, which can cause sex hormone changes. Over time, these chemicals can also cause inflammation—and, potentially, serious diseases.

Even supplements, which we give our children to be healthy, can contain ingredients that could cause a reaction. Cellulose, gelatin, food dyes, and natural flavorings are all vague descriptions and could contain GMOs or pesticides. The reaction to these mysterious ingredients, however, is not the problem. The reaction, usually a bumpy rash, should be a welcome warning signal. It is our body's way of telling us that inflammation is occurring. Left untreated, the inflammation can lead to stomach ulcers and disease. By "treating a reaction" I do not mean slapping a cream on it and hoping it will go away. I mean discovering the source of the problem and supporting the body to heal.

Avoiding toxic exposure and helping the gut to heal is crucial to any advances in health.

Something that a lot of parents often don't think of is that a child who frequently has a sign of food allergies, i.e. leaky gut or gut dysbiosis, or gets rashes, colds, or earaches fairly often, is likely to have a compromised immune system. Giving them medications and lotions may make things worse, not better. It is not unusual for such a child to react strongly to any medication, whether over the counter or prescribed. Your child with allergies is likely to be chemically sensitive as well, because his or her body is perceiving anything foreign as an invader (to protect itself) and the body's reaction can be severe. What's a parent to do? This is where many parents report in social media groups that alternative medicine has made a huge shift in their child or family's health. Integrative doctors, chiropractors, acupuncturists, iridologists, energy healers, detox clinics, oxygen therapy, and Chinese herbalists have been some of the alternatives that people have shared with me as their only source of true progress. Although Western medical doctors are imperative for some issues, many parents give up when their allopathic doctor doesn't find the cause of the problem but only treats the symptoms. I urge people not to give up and to try alternative methods. Ask other parents whose children have had the same health issues what worked for them. I promise you that even if your child has a rare disease, it is unfortunately not so rare any longer. Our children are sick. We need to stop trusting that the status quo treatments will make them better. We must use natural remedies and products, ask questions of our community, and take matters into our own hands with alternative doctors.

Vaccines

A new community that has formed with fervor and velocity is the health freedom or parental rights community. Just in the past few years, there has been an enormous new awareness of the possible dangers of vaccines.

One of the ways parents believe we are taking care of our children and preventing illness is to give them vaccines according to the CDC's schedule. Unfortunately, many parents do not consider that this schedule of forty-nine doses of vaccines by age twelve and sixty-nine doses by age eighteen could be harmful to their child. Nor do they read the list of ingredients or side effects on the package insert. Over the past few years, parents of vaccine damaged children have bravely come forward and are sharing their stories by the thousands through the movie and social media outlets of *VAXXED*, and in the docuseries *The Truth About Vaccines*, *Vaccines Revealed*, the movies *BOUGHT* and *Trace Amounts*. Every state now has a health freedom or parental rights Facebook group and numerous organizations have formed. The parents interviewed in these movies regret giving their babies five vaccine shots that contained multiple doses in each shot, when the baby was as young as three months old. They regret not reading the vaccine ingredients list and about the possible side effects.

When I began learning about GMOs and related pesticides, I began to get more and more friend requests on Facebook from health-minded mothers. One day a few years ago, a mother posted an image of the ingredients in vaccines. I had never read them before. My children were almost fully vaccinated. When I read the ingredients, some of which include thimerosal (mercury), aluminum, polysorbate 80, aborted fetal cells, and formaldehyde, I was deeply disturbed. Then I read bovine serum, fructose (sugar), soy, eggs, and dairy ingredients—and I knew these ingredients were likely GMO. I was even more disturbed. GMO ingredients, like soy and sugar in the vaccines or in food that was given to the livestock. Of the parts used in the vaccines, like bovine serum or eggs, many will likely contain not only DNA damaging GMOs but also glyphosate. This can wreak havoc on many functions of the body—particularly the gut, which is the stronghold of the immune system, and the brain.

I wondered . . . is glyphosate in vaccines? If so, can glyphosate herbicides be weakening the immune system and breaking down the blood-brain barrier, letting the toxins currently in the vaccines into the brain? In addition to the GMOs and toxins in my children's food, could glyphosate and toxins in vaccines have contributed to their litany of food allergies and autoimmune issues?

I thought about it and did some research. Although mercury has been identified as the leading cause of vaccine damage/autism, it began being added to vaccines in 1929 and there was no huge spike in autism then. In fact, the spike in autism happened in the late 1990s, just when glyphosate was introduced into the food supply via GMO foods. What if glyphosate herbicides were in vaccines and they were increasing the harmful impact of the toxins like mercury and aluminum, also in vaccines?

It cannot go unnoted, however, that just around the same time as the spike in autism, the number of vaccines required by the CDC increased as well, due to the National Childhood Vaccine Injury Act, which suddenly made vaccine manufacturers be free of any liability for the vaccines they produced. This meant that suddenly, no vaccine manufacturer could be sued for damage. This opened up the gates for vaccines to flood the market as they were suddenly without liability and therefore potentially much more lucrative. Parents of injured victims have to appeal to a special vaccine court, which has special judges, and is funded by a tax on vaccines. The tax is seventy-five cents per dose of each taxable vaccine, which is imposed on the manufacturer, and worked into the price that doctors pay for that vaccine. Manufacturers pay into this fund but don't have to be held accountable in court. Over $3.8 billion in awards to parents of vaccine damaged children have been paid out, clearly showing that vaccine damage exists, is real, and should be acknowledged by doctors and manufacturers.

Doctors, by the way, often get a financial incentive from the insurance companies for every child who is fully vaccinated if they meet a certain quota, so they have a financial motivation to have every child get vaccinated in their clinic and to "fire" patients who will not get vaccinated so that their percentages remain high. Most doctors dismiss claims that vaccines, with their current ingredients and at the current dosage, can be harmful because they simply do not know that they can be harmful. Many doctors have reported that the vaccine education they received in medical school was less than an hour and it was merely on how to administer them, not on the ingredients of the vaccines or their efficacy.

Although I knew it could be dangerous to my safety, as Dr. Bradstreet and nearly one hundred other doctors who spoke against traditional pharmaceutical products have been harassed or have been found dead by "suicide," I was highly motivated to get vaccines tested for glyphosate. Eventually, in 2016, I found a lab that agreed to test vaccines and I sent five childhood vaccines to be tested for glyphosate. I was shocked to learn that all five were positive. This meant that our children were, and likely still are, being injected with weed killer! Not only do these tests show that they are likely being injected with glyphosate, but very likely with the co-formulants in glyphosate-based herbicides as well, arsenic, petroleum-based chemicals, and heavy metals, which have been shown to be one thousand times more toxic than glyphosate alone! I was horrified. Truly horrified. I still am.

I learned from Seneff and Samsel that, in addition to GMO ingredients such as soy and sugar, glyphosate was most likely getting into vaccines through the GMO animal feed sprayed with glyphosate. The animals ate GMO grains, which can have levels up to 400 ppm of glyphosate. German scientist Monika Krueger has shown that glyphosate can collect in the bone marrow, tendons, and muscle tissue of animals. Several parts of the animals are used in vaccines. Specifically, the tendons of pigs are used to make gelatin, which is used to grow vaccines like MMR (measles, mumps, rubella) or to stabilize vaccines. It would make sense that gelatin, made of tendons, would therefore be high in glyphosate.

Our results showed that the MMR vaccine had glyphosate residues twenty-five times higher than the other vaccines—DTaP, pertussis, influenza, and pneumococcal. An independent scientist, Samsel, who followed up our testing and tested fourteen more vaccines for glyphosate showed that his MMR samples were thirty-four times higher than the other vaccines. This was fascinating because it was the MMR vaccine that Andy Wakefield, a former United Kingdom pediatric gastroenterologist, stated in a paper was connected to gut dysbiosis. He did not say the MMR caused autism, but children with autism have gut dysbiosis and there is an undeniable connection.

CDC whistleblower Dr. William Thompson has come forward and specifically said that the MMR vaccine caused higher rates of autism in children, especially African-American boys, and that the CDC knew this and covered it up for decades. In 2017, filmmaker Del Bigtree's nonprofit, Informed Consent Action Network (ICAN), sent a letter to the Department of Health and Human Services (which oversees the CDC) regarding vaccine safety. In the letter, they pointed out that Dr. Thompson, in a recorded phone call, stated the following regarding concealing this association: "Oh my God, I can't believe we did what we did. But we did. It's all there. It's all there. I have handwritten notes."

Dr. Thompson further stated on that call, "I have great shame now when I meet families with kids with autism because I have been part of the problem . . . the CDC is so paralyzed right now by anything related to autism. They're not doing what they should be doing because they're afraid to look for things that might be associated."

Andy Wakefield has been vilified, lost his license, and essentially lost his country—basically all because regulators are afraid to lose their jobs, and vaccine manufacturers don't want to lose their profits. William Thompson has still not been subpoenaed by congress. The cover-up continues.

I was sure however, that the finding of glyphosate in vaccines would cause scientists, doctors, the FDA, and the CDC to wonder if it was connected to the increase of vaccine related damage. After all, the spike in autism happened at the same time GMOs and glyphosate were introduced into our food, and therefore also into our vaccine supply. I was hoping that they would conduct testing and determine if this was the case. However, the FDA and the CDC both sent me letters claiming that vaccines are highly tested and safe. They did not answer my request for them to test for glyphosate in vaccines—or even mention it.

When I filed a Freedom of Information Act request a few months later, thinking that maybe they did test for glyphosate in vaccines but simply did not reveal the data, I received fifty-six pages back from the CDC that were over 50 percent redacted. They claimed that their "deliberative process" was protected. The documents that I received from the FDA were not redacted quite as much, but they left out eight months of the time period I requested. Clearly, both the CDC and the FDA were hiding something. Could this be because, according to Del Bigtree, the CDC holds twenty patents for vaccines and profits from their sales? Further pressure on our health agencies must be applied. Independent scientific research must be funded. In the meantime, parents must be educated in order to protect their children.

Educated moms like Rebecca Bredow, who during a custody battle went to jail in October 2017 for not following a court order to vaccinate her son, and Lori Matheson who faces the same judge in Detroit, Michigan, are both experiencing the sacrifice mothers must make to stand for their children's health in this new police state in which we are living. They face tens of thousands of dollars of legal bills, defamation, and even jail time. The court system is ignoring the fact that these mothers have a right to want to avoid injecting their children with ingredients found in vaccines such as aborted fetal tissues, cells of animals like pigs, cows, and hamsters, as well as numerous heavy metals and toxins. Mothers have reported having their children taken away from them by Child Protective Services or losing them in child custody cases to the fathers—all because they would not vaccinate. It is a tragedy. The children suffer because the lawyers convince the fathers that if they play the card of incompetent mother due to the lack of "care," i.e. vaccination, the father will win more or complete custody and therefore not have to pay as much or any child support. There is a group called American Divorce Association for Men or ADAM, based in Detroit, which uses these tactics in family law. This is a disgrace to our society.

It is truly essential that a solution be found to reverse the climbing rates of autism. Scientist Stephanie Seneff has done the calculations and she projects that if we continue at the current rate, by 2034 one out of two children born will have autism. Fifty percent of our children will be compromised! How will we function as a society? Who will fill our teacher positions? Our military? Our technology sector? Who will take care of their parents when they age? And from a political perspective—we will no longer be a world power if Americans are not able to realize their fullest potential!

It's not just our children who are being impacted by vaccines. Vaccine damage hit home when my ninety-one-year-old father went against my advice and got a high-dose flu shot in the fall of 2016. Before the shot, he had been taking long walks every day and only had the typical issues of aging—bad knees, macular degeneration, and bouts of prostate cancer that he was long recovered from. After the high-dose flu shot, within two months, he developed chronic kidney disease, emphysema, COPD, congestive heart failure, wheezing, and became unable to walk more than several feet without a walker. He had to have open-heart surgery. His 24-7 care cost him $12,000 a month. He now lives with my family and me, and after just a few months of his eating organic food and taking supplements, we reduced his medications from the eleven he was taking in the spring of 2017 down to two and a half (one he takes every other day) in the winter of 2017. We have seen significant improvements in his cognitive ability and wish that everyone knew about the risks of the high-dose flu shot. Dr. Joseph Mercola discusses these risks in his article, "Warn Your Friends and Family: The Fluzone High Dose Vaccine is Dangerous":

> According to the manufacturer's safety studies, compared to the regular Fluzone vaccine the high-dose version not only resulted in more frequent reports of common adverse reactions, it also caused slightly higher rates of Serious Adverse Events (SAE's).
>
> A total of 6.1 percent of seniors injected with the regular Fluzone vaccine experienced a serious adverse event, compared to 7.4 percent of those receiving the high-dose version.

When people try to imply that I am anti-vaccine for having tested vaccines for glyphosate, I simply respond that just like our food, vaccines are different now than they were when we were children. GMO chemical farming is contaminating almost everything: our corn, soy, wheat, beans, breast milk, wine, beer, cotton, feminine sanitary products—and yes, even vaccines.

There have been zero tests on the impact of glyphosate being injected into an infant or human of any age. Nor have there been any studies on the impact of glyphosate in conjunction with the other toxins in vaccines. Furthermore, Donna Farmer, lead toxicologist at Monsanto, admitted on the TV show *The Doctors* that glyphosate caused harm when it was injected into rats. However, she claimed that glyphosate is not administered that way (injected) in reality. Well, our reality has changed. And the fact is that no one, not our regulatory agencies, the manufacturers, nor your doctor, can accurately claim that any vaccines as they are currently formulated, containing glyphosate herbicides, are safe.

To find out more about vaccines I suggest going to www.nvic.org, the website of the National Vaccine Information Center.

> The journey to empowerment is often one you never imagined. It can start in misery, despair, tragic loss, and the daily struggle with the incomprehensible impact of vaccine damage. But when we are willing to listen to honest, hurting parents, and heed their warnings . . . we get the courage that it takes to tell one's story. We connect with a stranger. We are empowered to take action that we otherwise might not have taken, like being brave in the doctor's office and refusing to vaccinate our own children with five shots containing ten diseases and multiple toxins in one sitting. Those connections, and acts of bravery, are happening across the country and are actually saving lives. Unity based on tragedy is empowering.

Protecting Our Animals

It's not just our human children that are likely being impacted by toxins. Our pets and wildlife are being harmed as well. Have you noticed an increase of tumors in dogs? Does your cat struggle with anxiety? Did your pet die earlier than was expected? Have you heard of the increase of heart attacks in racehorses on the tracks? There are many factors that are contributing to this tragic increase of animal sickness and death including food, environmental factors, and vaccines. The amount of toxins in pet and livestock vaccines is not an area that many have researched, but some veterinarians—such as Dr. John Robb, a thirty-year veterinarian in Connecticut who lost his clinic from fighting the vaccine schedule, particularly for rabies—say that vaccines are the cause of harm and death. He reported to government officials that small dogs who received the same doses of the rabies vaccine as large dogs often died. To keep our pets and animals safe, we must reduce their toxic burden.

Food is the most consistent contributor to an animal's health. Unfortunately, the pet owner community and animal advocates can no longer just trust the label on a pet food package, even if it says "natural." In general, the safety standards and requirements to disclose ingredients are far less rigorous for animal food than human food. Many ingredients do not have to be disclosed, and many euphemisms can be used for some of the unhealthiest ingredients.

According to Slate.com's Jackson Landers, from his article "A Dog-Eat-Dog-World":

> There is essentially no federal enforcement of standards for the contents of pet food. Officially the FDA has authority, but the agency has passed off regulating the standards to nongovernmental organizations that encourage mostly voluntary compliance with the few federal standards.

Under Food and Drug Administration regulations, only about 50 percent of a cow, for instance, can be sold for human consumption. The hide, bones, digestive system and its contents, brain, feces, udders, and various other undesirable parts, are all left over after a cow is slaughtered and butchered. The stuff that can't even go into hot dogs gets consolidated and shipped to rendering plants.

Personally, I do not have a problem with my dogs eating the "undesirable parts" of animals. In the wild, they would have eaten anything that they could break down with their teeth, which would have been almost everything. There would have been one exception, however—they would not eat meat that was rotten or diseased. They could sense it and they would leave the carcass to be picked at by vultures and insects.

Today, however, according to animal rights activists, animals are fed food that could easily be rotten or diseased—including meat from other cats and dogs, roadkill, and expired grocery store meat still in the Styrofoam packaging. Of course, they are also eating unregulated meat from animals fed GMO grains with a vast array of pesticide, herbicide, and fungicide residues.

Pet foods such as Purina brands, Friskies, Kibbles 'n Bits, 9 Lives, Rachael Ray Nutrish, and Iams brands have been tested positive for glyphosate weed killer and its breakdown AMPA at levels from .065 ppb to .24 ppb. Glyphosate bioaccumulates in bone marrow, so any amount is concerning. There should be zero glyphosate herbicide and toxins in our pets' food. It is simply animal cruelty to feed our pets poison.

What can we do? This is a tricky one. Most Americans feel they cannot afford to feed their pets organic food—with good reason, since it is significantly more expensive than nonorganic. However, most people feed their pets far too much food, and as a result our pets are overweight. You might switch to organic food, which has been shown to be more nutritious than regular pet food, and therefore not as much food will be needed. You can feed your pet less, find that they are healthier on a more reasonable budget, and save on future veterinary costs as well.

Website resources Dog Food Advisor and Modern Farmer suggest that pet owners buy organic food sourced from animals that are humanely raised. If that isn't possible, they suggest the following:

> Buy the most natural pet food you can and add in your leftover, diced-up scraps. Dogs that eat vegetables mixed into their dog food get 70 percent less heart attacks. Chop up your salad scraps, vegetable stems or tops and add them to your pet's food. Pets need their veggies, too! You can also reduce or eliminate commercial dog food by feeding your dog "human" food—just be careful. There are many human foods dogs should not eat, such as grapes, raisins, chocolate, and cooked poultry bones (raw are okay). Butchers will often give you leftover meat, bone, or fat scraps for free if you tell them you are feeding it to your dog. Cook them up (to kill any possible parasites) with a little Himalayan Pink salt for minerals and your pet will be thrilled.

Other livestock animals such as goats and horses are being impacted by the subpar animal feed standards as well. GMO grains and nonorganic forage that livestock and horses eat are commonly sprayed with glyphosate as a drying agent in order to speed up the harvesting process. In May 2013, the EPA raised the allowable levels of glyphosate residues, for instance, on corn from 2 ppm to 13 ppm. Suddenly in 2014, animals eating these grains could have been eating six to three hundred times more glyphosate herbicide residues than in previous feeds. A farmer who sent GMO Roundup Ready alfalfa for testing reported to me positive results for over 19,000 ppb of glyphosate. At the same time, reports of increased deaths on racetracks were reported and veterinarians reported a sharp rise in tumors in animals. Owners of GMO-fed goats and pigs report their livestock produce less milk than in previous years. Birth defects, smaller litters, and deaths of young livestock have repeatedly been shown to rise in animals fed GMO and glyphosate sprayed grains. This practice is inhumane animal abuse and must be stopped.

I was glad to learn that animal activists prevailed in Utah in June 2017, when the courts decided that a proposed law to ban the filming of factory farms was a violation of free speech. In some states, an employee/undercover activist can still record the practices inside a factory farm and release it to the public.

This form of accountability is very effective in compelling farmers who raise animals to treat them humanely. It is also very compelling to consumers, helping convince them to switch from conventional meat to no meat at all. These choices greatly impact the meat industry, encouraging more and more farmers to reconsider their practices and treat animals with respect and kindness. Some grow diverse vegetable crops instead, reducing the amount of both carbon and toxins released into the environment.

> If you or a loved one want to learn more about factory farming, one way is to share the fictional but true to life book *Toxin* by Robin Cook. Another idea is to watch *Vegucated, What the Health, Forks Over Knives,* or *Okja* to raise awareness with your family or friends. Be gentle, not judgmental, when you share information about factory farming and veganism, and people will be much more receptive, grateful, and open to making changes.

Wildlife such as birds, insects, moose, and more are being terribly impacted by toxins. Glyphosate and other toxins used in farming are also used in "conservation" efforts in the wilderness to "protect" native species. California fisheries reported a 70 percent drop in fish populations in 2015. A 2017 Canadian report showed that over half of Canada's monitored wildlife is in decline, with the declining species having lost *83 percent of their population.* Monarch butterflies are disappearing, and even the rain is showing levels of herbicides. Our bees have experienced a 30 to 90 percent die-off in some areas. In October 2017, a study from Germany revealed a 75 percent die-off over three decades of the insect population *in a nature reserve* around pesticide sprayed farms. The frightening thing to consider is that history shows that we have been through five mass extinctions on our planet. Through all five, insects have survived. If we are killing off our insects at this rate, what future do we humans have? The massive decline of songbird populations is already being attributed to the loss of insects and presence of toxic chemicals. The health and environmental crisis from the impact on this planet of the poisoning from toxic chemicals is real. If we don't do something fast, the world our grandchildren will grow up in—if our children are able to conceive—will be one devoid of most of the wonders of nature that we have enjoyed.

Many conservation groups have been convinced to use herbicides to fend off invasive weeds and therefore use Roundup and other toxic chemicals in millions of acres of parks and wilderness. With the stacks of new studies piling up however, the concept that the hundreds of millions of pounds of herbicides and pesticides that are aerially sprayed over forests and fields are actually contributing to the decline of wildlife can no longer be ignored. Many studies have shown that these chemicals are endocrine disruptors, meaning that they can cause sterility and harm or halt the development of a fetus, leading to the decline of a population.

Marine life is also being impacted as our rivers and oceans are being polluted. For example, the sea turtles off the coast of Maui are riddled with cancerous tumors from the fertilizer and pesticide run-off. A 2011 report stated, 85 percent of the world's oyster beds have disappeared due to overfishing and disease which can be exacerbated by the presence of immune system weakening chemicals like glyphosate.

Our salmon are now being genetically modified to grow four times fatter, four times faster, and to be sterile. We raise them in tanks with antibiotics and hormones and feed them GMO fish food. The GM salmon are aggressive and could wipe out wild salmon. Somewhere along the line, our disconnection with nature allowed some people to bring about a dramatic manipulation and pollution of nature without the rest of us noticing. For twenty years, chemical companies have been altering our food supply and spraying chemicals on our food and soil with impunity. Scientist Rosemary Mason has described in detail how we are currently in the sixth mass extinction. There is no way back for some species, she says—we have poisoned ourselves for too long. I myself must hope that there is still something we can do.

Despite our losses of wilderness preserves and wildlife, and the lack of bans on chemicals and GMO regulation, I am clear that with every breakdown, there is an opportunity for a breakthrough. What's happening is a massive breakdown for life on the planet, and therefore a massive breakthrough is possible if we take the necessary actions, leadership and political will.

Guilt, Blame, and Anger

One of the most common responses that I see when people learn about GMOs and toxins in human food, pet food, and other products, besides anger and confusion, is guilt. For nine years, I fed my son GMOs and did not know the ramifications. I didn't read the ingredient lists of body care products, vaccines, or most foods, and I regret that. When I realized what my lack of knowledge and inaction might have done to my child, I was racked with guilt. Guilt equals stress, which can actually lead to sickness and disease. I felt my body weaken and I knew I would get sick if I continued to focus on the past. So, I decided to take an objective look at the situation and ask myself, how could I have known? The FDA didn't tell us that Monsanto quietly started supplying farmers with GMO crops, hoping that things would stay under the radar and no one would notice. No one in my family knew about this. None of my close friends, the media, or any teachers told me about GMOs for nine years. Not even my doctor knew! No one. So, I began to shift away from blaming myself. Because when you know better, you do better. I just didn't know before. That doesn't mean I was a bad mom. I just didn't know. How could I? How could you?

> Don't allow yourself to cop out or blame and distance others. Plug in. Take action. And invite the person that you want to support to take action, too, in a lighthearted, fun, and loving way. Life will be easier and more fulfilling, and you will feel more powerful.

Once I did know better and started taking action, then there was the guilt about not being as effective as I would like. Guilt seemed to be triggered by sources all around me outside the home. How could my neighbor with Parkinson's still be using Roundup after all the flyers I had dropped off and conversations we have had about it? What was I doing wrong? How could I be a better neighbor?

Feeling guilty about not doing something well enough is ineffective in several ways. Taking on the responsibility of other people's choices is a form of belittling them. Think about it. By blaming ourselves, we are actually saying that what happens to them is *our* fault. We have the power. We end up taking away their power and seeing them as small.

On the other hand, blaming others for not knowing about the harm that could come to them or their families from not avoiding toxins is also not productive. Too often I see on social media comments like, "Idiot!" "Sheeple!" or "Get your head out of the sand!" I am going to pull the mom card and say *be nice*. People do not listen to people who are angry with them, blame them, belittle them, or make them feel even slightly wrong for what they eat or how they care for their children. When I get angry with someone, I try to remember that I didn't know, either, at one time.

Feeling guilty about the lack of progress, or the delay of it, and blaming others only accomplishes three things:

1. It disempowers you.
2. It disempowers others.
3. It delays growth and progress.

I am not suggesting that you set aside your belief that you *can* make a difference with others, because you can. Catch yourself if guilt about the situation turns into flippant dismissal. If you start thinking, "Well, they are going to do whatever they want, anyway," get that that is resignation and doubt. Catch it. Don't give up if change doesn't happen quickly—but also don't blame yourself if change doesn't happen quickly, either.

Or, are you angry about what is going on in the world? Is it exhausting you and making you feel sick? I would say that your anger is correlated to how much you care. I might even say it's causational. (If you didn't care, you would not be mad.) Focus on how much you care, what you care about, and be glad that you care! Spend time with your kids, family, and pets. Get in touch with your community. Spend time talking to your neighbors about

Roundup. Enjoy being with them. Enjoy going to city council meetings and connecting with city policy makers. Then the anger will dissipate, you will be healthier . . . and you will be able to take on the world.

Celebrate Community

People have asked me how I keep going and don't burn out. My answer is to acknowledge and celebrate the people who have dedicated themselves to our cause. Nothing inspires me more than getting connected to the generous and committed people who are also taking action for health and freedom.

On December 10, 2015, Organic Consumers Association organized the DARK (Denying Americans the Right to Know) Act rally in Washington, DC. Sponsors paid for busloads of people to show up at the senate hearing in which GMO labeling would be discussed. People came from all across the country. It was thrilling. The hearing did not turn out as we had hoped, however. The security guards in the senate halls wouldn't even let us sit while we waited for hours to get into the hearing because sitting was seen as an act of protest, and for that one could be arrested. We were blocked by law students who admitted to being paid to be in line (presumably by GMO proponents) hours ahead of time and prevented the entry of most of our people. After flying across the country from California to be there, I was three people away from getting into the hearing. I watched the hearing on my phone outside the courtroom and fumed.

To our horror, one of our own, Scott Faber the vice president of government affairs of the Environmental Working Group and executive director of the nonprofit Just Label It, who was testifying, stated that, "No one is seeking a ban on GMOs," and "We do not oppose . . . genetically modified food ingredients. We think there are many promising applications of genetically modified food ingredients . . . I am optimistic that the promises that were made by the providers of this technology will ultimately be realized . . . that we will have traits that produce more nutritious food that will see significant yield."

When asked if GMOs were as safe as their conventional counterparts, he answered, "Yes."

After this shocking betrayal, several hundred activists gathered at a nearby church. I felt like I had been punched in the chest until I saw the friendly faces of people from Michigan, Florida, Pennsylvania, Massachusetts, and beyond. I recognized them from years of social media interaction. We whooped with joy, hugged, laughed, and exclaimed how happy we were to finally meet each other. My heart was truly full. I was honored to be introduced to their delightful children, who also hugged me, and to hold their hands with gratitude. Together, we ate organic, vegan, delicious food and talked about our next steps. It was a true celebration of community. Not because we had succeeded at the day's efforts, but because by gathering together, we had deepened our faith that in the long run we would prevail.

> Being the one to say, "Let's get together," and inviting your local community to learn about the issues, discuss them, and eat healthy food while you meet each other, builds relationships. These gatherings are essential for having you—both you individually, and you and your group collectively—be UNSTOPPABLE. Take that time to acknowledge and celebrate each other.

Because we are a movement of social connections and sharing knowledge, when the Food Justice Rally organizers in Washington, DC, and Moms Across America in California gave out awards to notable leaders, doctors, lawyers, and activists, collectively, the people of the movement felt acknowledged.

> Celebrating each other fuels the movement onward and upward. Feeling burned out? Take a moment to call or write a note to a friend or fellow activist and thank him or her for doing something that inspired you. Thank your spouse, kids, or family for being open to the information you have to share or for buying organic food and, as a result, you will feel revitalized.

PART THREE

UNSTOPPABLE LEADERSHIP

CHAPTER SEVEN
ACTIVISM

"Our lives begin to end the day we become silent about things that matter."
—MARTIN LUTHER KING, JR.

ONCE I HAD found my tribe, my community, people that understood and could commiserate with me, I eventually exhausted my need for commiserating. Instead of talking, I wanted to actually *do* something. I wanted to make a difference. I wanted to not only heal my kids and my friend's kids, I wanted to transform the food industry so that no one's children, regardless of their income or location, would be subjected to poisons and harm.

Doing something meant stepping outside my comfort zone, however—not an easy thing to do for a mom who already has enough to do. But soon I learned the incredible power of stepping into a role of leadership, no matter what kind: in your family, school, town, community, or country.

Empowerment in Action

I admit that I once thought that activists were fussbudgets who had too much time on their hands. I looked down on them, pitied them, and was even repelled by them. I thought for sure they smelled of patchouli and would ramble on forever about ice caps and whales if I got too close. I steered clear of the Greenpeace people outside of grocery stores even though I fundamentally agreed with everything they stood for—protecting life on the planet.

Over the years, my thinking has changed, and so has society's. Activism has once again been embraced by a vocal majority of people of all ages who care about issues such as human rights, animal rights, election integrity, and environmental rights.

Civil rights, women's right to vote, unions, child labor laws, and more all have made strides (albeit not enough) through activism. Nations have been formed and humans have been freed due to the impassioned efforts of activists. They were not paid. They were not promised anything. They did what they did because they saw a need for justice. Many times, they failed or fell short, but in many cases, justice prevailed.

Activism has been perceived by nonactivists as ineffectual because their actions are often not highlighted by the media. It does not serve the mainstream news outlets to feature activists who are thwarting the power and profits of major corporations that foot the bill of the television network. No, that would be biting the hand that feeds you.

You have to wonder—when millions of people in over four hundred cities march against the corruption of our government by one of the largest chemical companies in the world, Monsanto, and it doesn't make the news—isn't someone making sure the story doesn't get told?

You have to wonder—when thirty thousand doctors in Argentina file a petition to ban glyphosate, why isn't that in the news in the United States?

> Being an activist means being willing to accept the hard truth. It means looking for the truth and being skeptical about what you are being served up by the media and the government and then asking hard questions. Being an activist means doing your own research, talking with people who are affected by the issue, and taking action to support justice. It is simply what you do if you care about something.

Vani Hari, *New York Times* bestselling author and founder of FoodBabe.com says:

> When I dedicated my life to being a food activist I knew the fight was going to be long and difficult—but I never knew how much I'd learn about handling detractors who don't want us to succeed. We've helped change multi-billion-dollar food and beverage companies for the better and this has come with great resistance. When I started to get personally attacked, one of my dear mentors said, "Did you think the powerful chemical companies and food giants of the world were going to let us waltz right into their

world and turn it upside down?" Hearing this put perspective on the impact we are making as activists. If you do things that are remarkable, people are going to remark and if they fight back, it means you are winning.

Our Role As Americans

There is a new definition of what it means to be "a proud American." Many of us are seeing that it no longer means we trust our government implicitly and stand behind its decisions with patriotic fervor. Being a proud American means standing up for the rights and freedoms that those who came before us fought so hard to win, even if we face adversity and scorn. It means researching, thinking for ourselves, getting to the truth, and going against the grain of convenience and popular perceptions. Deliberate ignorance does not serve us . . . nor future generations.

One stay-at-home mom who learned about the harsh reality of our food system and spoke up to protect her family and country was Tami Canal, the initiator of the March Against Monsanto. In her own words, Tami summarizes the importance of the movement:

> I started March Against Monsanto (MAM) as a response to the failure of Prop 37, a 2012 ballot initiative in California. Prop 37 would have simply required the labeling of all foods made with genetically modified ingredients. It was a very straightforward initiative that would have allowed people to know what was in the food they were buying. Unfortunately, big industries like Monsanto, DuPont, and Nestle funneled millions into the pro-corporation/anti-citizen choice outcome.
>
> I knew that I had started making better choices at the grocery store such as choosing organic and opting out of the GMO experiment. I realized that if more people knew what was happening that they too would make better choices in spending their money at the store. I decided to start a Facebook page that included a global call to action. The global call to action was about getting people in the streets, handing out information, and educating their communities because I believe when people know better, they do better. The first March Against Monsanto (MAM) on

May 25, 2013, saw more than two million people in more than four hundred cities get out into the streets to protest Monsanto and the corporate hijack of both the food supply and our planet.

The first MAM far exceeded my original goals of having three thousand people join in. The incredible turnout for that first march was due largely in part to the signing of The Monsanto Protection Act (which has since been repealed) in March 2013 when President Obama signed legislation that granted Monsanto complete judicial immunity—meaning that if a product made by Monsanto made someone sick, there was no recourse for that person to sue Monsanto. People were rightfully enraged by such an unconstitutional act and March Against Monsanto gave them an outlet to channel that outrage into productivity by raising community awareness.

Although I am very proud of the awareness that MAM has raised globally, I am most proud of witnessing the development of community leadership that MAM has spawned. Stay-at-home moms, college students, people who had never been to a protest stepped up to lead their cities. These inspiring individuals have changed the course of history and it is an amazing feeling to know that the March Against Monsanto lit that spark that ignited a global movement.

It is powerful and thrilling to reach millions of people in a single day, whether through social media, marches, or parades. The energy at my local March Against Monsanto in Laguna Beach, California, with over one thousand people, was electrifying. We have seven billion people on the planet, however, and many still do not know about the harmful effects of GMOs or toxic chemicals. In the United States, we face a particularly daunting situation because 85 to 100 percent of our major crops such as corn, soy, and sugar beets are now GMO. How did it get this way? We simply did not know it was happening . . . and we did not act. In Europe, however, when the media reported that scientist Arpad Pusztai discovered that rats that ate GMO potatoes had severe health issues, GMO crops were banned within weeks and EU grocery stores required the labeling of all GMO ingredients. GMOs are simply not grown or wanted in most of Europe, due to health concerns. I was thrilled to have the opportunity to go to Europe and be a part of an international protest over a small plot of GMO potatoes in the countryside.

It was a sunny Saturday in Switzerland. We started out on a storybook picturesque farm valley east of Zurich with a van full of speakers and activists. We drove for nearly an hour to the outskirts of Zurich to start the rally at a typically Swiss, tree-lined square. The International Demonstration Against Corporate Control and GMOs (August 22, 2015) had been denied access to the center of Zurich and from gathering at the research facility. It didn't stop them. Our host Urs Hans was a down-to-earth man, an activist and farmer, well known in his region. A few years earlier, he had realized that his fellow farmers' calves were dying shortly after vaccinations. He refused to vaccinate his calves and it resulted in a standoff between him and the government that rallied farmers from far and wide. For the first time ever, differences between varying types of farmers—mountain farmers and valley farmers, conventional and ecological, poor and wealthy, cattle, goat and sheep farmers—were set aside. All came together to fight against mandatory vaccinations of their animals. Urs and the farmers won. Their animals did not die of the disease that the government proclaimed would wipe out the livestock.

Urs was UNSTOPPABLE in his stand for his animals, and I am pretty sure that is why he related to my speech when he saw me speak in Denver, Colorado, at the "Seeds of Doubt" conference. When a Moms Across America supporter, Nadia Negro, heard Urs asking me questions, she recognized his accent and said to him in Swiss German, "We need to talk." She was moving back to her homeland, Switzerland, and she said, "I want to keep going—we have to do something." She, too, was UNSTOPPABLE. The two of them got together in Switzerland and organized an event for myself and several international speakers to address their citizens at a demonstration against corporate control and the test-planting of GMO potatoes in their region.

This may sound like just another rally, but it really was extraordinary on so many levels. First, Switzerland does not cultivate GMO crops, it does not import or feed their livestock GMOs, and it does not allow GMOs in Swiss food—either made locally or imported. GMOs are not a part of their daily life. To ask anyone to protest something which is not impacting them, and to have nearly one thousand people show up, is true dedication—and, I must say, sheer brilliance on everyone's part.

Second, the test plot was a mere few hundred feet of a fenced-in field of potatoes, something that would not cause most people to even blink an eye. It would not be on the news, since it was not planted near a school or church.

It looked harmless. To have so many people march from the outskirts of town through Zurich and back out through a small village to this potato field was a feat most Americans would not think possible.

Third, the moratorium preventing GMOs from being grown for industry in the EU would not expire until 2017. (The activists were successful in getting the ban extended to 2021.) At the time, the expiration was nearly *two years* in the future. Most people don't plan a month out—never mind plan a protest for something that will not truly impact them for another two years. The organizers and their families and friends were truly dedicated people. Everyone who showed up and marched in the bright sun passed out flyers, chanted, and sang and danced down the streets of Zurich and small villages for hours are truly extraordinary people. But in Europe, they see this as just ordinary. It's just what they do.

I love America, and yet being in Switzerland and seeing the dedication of the activists left me wondering about the American mindset. One of the protesters, a young man wearing a potato sack, asked me curiously, "Why aren't Americans doing more about this? Why are they letting GMOs be planted everywhere? Why don't they do something?"

I was reminded of an article I saw posted on Facebook in which a person suggested that the fluoride in our water could be connected to complacency. It was put into the water of prison camps, the article stated, and made the prisoners docile, passive, and easier to manage. Such a theory is unproven . . . but one must wonder . . . why is fluoride in our water if Harvard University studies have found it to be a neurotoxin? Could it be making us more complacent? Why aren't Americans more active about stopping GMOs and pesticides from polluting our country and harming our children? Or is it just that the media didn't tell us because they are controlled by Big Pharma?

I told the man that unfortunately, for seventeen years, I did not know about GMOs. The media did not tell us about them. The only reason I realized GMOs were harmful is that my children got sick. Most Americans don't know—or if they know but aren't sick, they don't care. They don't have reason to care . . . until they or a loved one gets sick.

I grapple with this still. I now know thousands of activists and supporters who do care and go to extraordinary lengths to raise awareness. I am enlivened and inspired by them. The switch has turned *on* for millions due to efforts from people like Tami, and there is no turning it off. I wonder every day how we can support more people to turn their switches to *on*. How can we raise awareness with hundreds of millions—or billions—of people so that they realize what is happening and are compelled to do anything and everything they can to stop it? My only answer for now is through empowerment and love.

A Native American Mother Sparks an International Movement

Empowerment and love were definitely present when a mom, LaDonna Brave Bull Allard, realized that the oil companies planned to run a pipeline through, Standing Rock and risk polluting the Sioux Nation ancestral burial grounds where her son was buried. In addition, the pipeline would likely poison her reservation's only water supply, so she made a call to stop the oil companies.

Within weeks, Americans from all different backgrounds descended upon Standing Rock in droves to protect indigenous rights and the water from being polluted, which would impact eighteen million people downstream. Seeing this as a community issue and wanting to protect against the further poisoning of any people, Moms Across America supporters rallied and asked me to go and bring supplies. They wanted MAA to stand with the women, young warriors, elderly, and men who were peacefully protecting their water, land, and rights. I did. Our supporters gave over $10,000, allowing us to donate wood and supplies for their survival during the harsh winter. When we arrived at the camp, which had flags from an unprecedented 300 native tribes lining the Crazy Horse main road, we were mesmerized by the utopia, in a sense, of community. Complete strangers would walk up to people building a teepee and help out. We were offered pumpkin soup just because we were walking by. My sons chopped firewood for hours beside a Sioux woman as a young man scraped a deer hide (roadkill) nearby. They shaved the bark off logs for a yurt to be used as a medic tent until their hands were caked with birch sap. We helped in the kitchens, art camp, and building of structures. We attended daily morning community meetings that opened with prayer, song, sage, and ceremony. All people were treated with dignity and respect.

When the peaceful demonstration on Sunday, November 20, 2016 turned violent, and I was among those teargassed on the bridge, people were blasted with flash grenades, mace, and tear gas, and elders were drenched with freezing water, I almost lost my faith in humanity. It was heartbreaking to see young people fall to the ground, shot in the back of the legs with rubber bullets, for guarding a fire from being extinguished that was keeping them from getting hypothermia. But when droves of the Water Protectors arrived to carry them to the infirmary, others arrived to take their place, and even more gave the drenched people new donated coats, handed them soup, and washed mace off their faces, I felt hope again. The people of the community took care of each other.

Being at Standing Rock, I was reminded of the decency of people, the UNSTOPPABLE love of mothers, the honor we need to give our elderly, and the wisdom and tenacity of the youth—which can literally save the world. Indigenous leaders around the world are now coming together to sign declarations to protect the earth.

Standing Rock was the beginning of a new, worldwide revolution of community involvement to protect our water, land, health, and freedom. When the media covered the November 20th activist event—because it was obviously a valid cause, just, urgent, and unfortunately, violent—suddenly, some activists actually felt hope. Over 300 people were injured that night and the violence was devastating, but the fact that peaceful demonstrations caused President Obama to stop the pipeline and led to coverage in the international media, lawsuits, and eventually a judgment in the activists' favor, gave new life to activism everywhere.

Standing Rock was not necessarily a cause that MAA originally set out to focus on, but when your community expands, so does your action plan. Often, groups tend to myopically focus on one thing. What we realized by participating in this event was that we all want the same things: namely, clean water, air, food, medicines, healthy families, justice, and freedom.

> Driving to another state or flying across the country might not work for you right now. Start with your family. If you want to go beyond being a leader in your own family, step out into your neighborhood, school, church, county, or state. There are people and organizations to help you along the way. Our global community needs you, your unique abilities, your perspective, and your love.

How to Get Involved

People ask us at Moms Across America every day, "How do I get involved? How can I volunteer? What do I do?"

The best way to get involved is to *invite others to get involved*. Share. You can post an existing event such as an Earth Day Fair or Independence Day Parade on social media or create a new event like a Healthy Kids Park Playdate and invite people to get together. Once you gather, after getting acquainted and having fun together, you can decide how to take action as a group to protect your community.

There are so many fun things you can do to raise awareness and strengthen your community, such as hosting a movie night, a tea, or a garden share (share surplus food from your garden). Or invite friends over to make soap, kefir cheese, or sauerkraut . . . whatever is most fun for you. I was delighted to learn that MAA supporters and leaders of GMO Free Lancaster County started a monthly "skill share" where members of the group took turns teaching each other skills like installing solar or growing sprouts. Once connected, as a group, you can go to your school board or city council and have them stop spraying Roundup. You could approach your school food director to have more organic food served at your school (check out TurningGreen.org and their Conscious Kitchen Project). You could even buddy up to create a community garden!

If you post an event on MomsAcrossAmerica.org, other local people can connect with you. You can also get a code for a free box of flyers from MAA to empower your community.

Drop a stack of one hundred flyers off at your library, schools, churches, chiropractors, and senior centers! Leaving flyers at a gas station in the travel brochure section, in a hotel in the tourists' flyer boxes, or in a doctor's office magazine rack—*stealth activism*—can make a difference for someone you will never even meet.

If you have a movie night and ten people come, give each person a stack of 100 flyers (do *not* let them just take two or three), then ask them if they will leave these at their schools, churches, libraries, grocery stores, and farmers markets. If each flyer inspires a new family to spend $100 a week on organic food, then in one week you and your friends will have created a $5 million shift to organic per year for your neighborhood. If each one of those people who got a flyer then convinces five of their friends to buy $100 a week of organic food, then you have created a $26 million shift per year in your community! With ten friends, that's over $50 million!

If only fifty-six people in each state in America would do this, we would double the sales of organic, from $50 billion in sales to $100 billion, reduce toxic exposure, support organic farming, and reduce the greenhouse gases that impact climate change in America!

Don't you think that would make a big difference for our local organic farmers and our community's health? I do!

Your actions make a difference! We can create healthy communities together now!

Time

When people consider volunteering, or getting involved in activism, I am often told, "I just don't have the time right now." Here's the rub—we all have the same amount of time and we all make choices on what to do with that time. The problem is that those choices may not align with what really matters to us.

When you find something that is truly important to you, how do you fit it into your life? Spending time on things that give our life meaning and value—and benefit others as well—are actions worth making time for. Everyone can find time in his or her week. Can you forego that television show, or combine flyer distribution with your evening run? Can you drop off a stack of flyers at the library while your children return their books? If you are spending your time stressing over the high cost of medical bills, stop stressing and take action in your home that will likely reduce—or possibly even eliminate—your medical expenses. I believe you will find much greater satisfaction in doing something like making healthy organic food at home on Sundays, cleaning out your toxic household cleaners, or asking the city council to stop spraying toxic chemicals in your town on a Tuesday evening.

> The trick to managing your time is to ask yourself, what is most important to me in the long term? What can I do right now about that? Put it in your calendar, make time to do it, and then don't let anything dissuade you.

Money

I didn't have the money to start Moms Across America when I started it. However, I was determined to start it, and keep doing it, regardless of whether I had two pennies to rub together or not. Why? Because it mattered that much to me. It still does. That commitment and determination is what got me the money to make it happen.

You may want to pass out flyers at a city festival, bring organic snacks to a community event, or start a school garden, but may not have the money to do it. Don't ever let money stop you.

I didn't have the two thousand dollars to start a website, so I asked for it, and got it. The trick to raising money is that there is no trick. You must be authentic, honest, passionate, and completely clear about what you are doing. If you want seeds and soil for the school garden, ask the nursery for a donation or do a bake sale to raise the funds. If you want money for flyers or snacks for a school event, ask the local health food store for a donation. I hosted a "Moms Night In to Boot Toxins Out" party at my home, where we made sauerkraut, and my local health food store gave me a fifty-dollar gift card to buy healthy, organic snacks for the event . . . because I asked for it. Many times, people are happy to give if you just ask.

> When fundraising, make sure to communicate in a way that makes a difference for others—what is in it for them? What results will they see that will benefit their goals? How will you spend the money? How many people will you reach and what difference will that make? Ask for what you need. Need fifty dollars or $100,000? It's the same conversation. Just ask. If you are clear about your goals, have a project that will make a difference, and you are authentic in how you ask for it, money will not be a problem. It will come.

The Toxin-Free Town Campaign

I grew up in a small town in Connecticut amid green, rolling hills, state forest land, and plentiful rivers, streams, and lakes. My childhood home had a beautiful, private pond teeming with life. Skate bugs skimmed the surface, water snakes, purple flowering reeds, shiny black-backed turtles, smallmouth bass, and great blue herons were daily sightings.

This is the pond that my father asked my brother, sister, and me to pull the weeds from when I was a child. This is the pond where I, at the age of twelve, told my father we should dump Roundup into instead, to kill the weeds.

"No," he said definitively. His no resonated deep in his throat—a place from which no reversal was possible.

I persisted anyway. I hated pulling the weeds. The muck from the bottom of the pond would rise to the surface, swirl around my body, coating my body hairs and leaving me covered in pond scum.

"But Dad, it's safe . . . They said so on TV." Commercials for Roundup said it was safe and effective! I was frustrated that he refused to believe that modern technology could actually be useful. *Stubborn old goat.* He would rather use his children as slave labor. I didn't realize at the time that my father was the first environmentalist that I encountered.

"No," he said again. "It will kill the frogs."

I groaned, still disbelieving. Little did I know that I would devote my life to ridding the planet of Roundup and other toxic chemicals thirty years later.

Today I know better—many of us know better. Groups of citizens, often led by moms, have asked their towns to discontinue the use of Roundup and toxic chemicals and have been successful. Chicago, Illinois, Boulder, Colorado, Portland, Maine, and Marin County, Irvine, Mission Viejo, and Burbank, California are just some of the communities that have discontinued the use of Roundup around water reservoirs, or some—or all—streets and parks.

One day Natalie Paffrath, a mom, nurse, and our MAA board treasurer who lives in my town, called me, furious, and said that a truck with a tank had just sprayed her street with Rodeo (a glyphosate-based herbicide). She had a picture of the truck spraying. That day, we filed a complaint with the county agricultural commissioner and went to the Orange County Public Works with a binder of studies. After one meeting and a few calls and emails, the manager agreed to propose alternatives. Since then, our city has agreed to stop spraying glyphosate-based herbicides in residential neighborhoods. Due to the efforts of many committed parents, my son's entire school district has also agreed to use alternatives such as safer chemicals, mulch, and weed whacking. This was especially important to me because we noticed that Bodee would have trouble breathing, and had asthma symptoms, after the city workers had sprayed Roundup on the hillsides by his school. It is terrifying to see your child having difficulty breathing. I am so grateful that his school district has discontinued the use of glyphosate herbicides.

In a *Chicago Tribune* article in September 2017, Meg Hegarty wrote:

> Meg Torres, a Naperville, Illinois resident and avid gardener, signed a petition to eliminate Roundup use in her town and believes using Roundup is an "old way of doing things. We need to do better, we need to find an alternative and be an example for other towns and cities when it comes to managing our landscape," Torres said. "Most people are concerned about what this does to monarch butterflies and honeybees, but for me it's my kids, they're the most important thing."

This Illinois citizen's initiative was a success!

How Do You Have Your Town Go Toxin-Free?

Although it may seem like a daunting task, the reality is that many people have had their city or school district discontinue the use of toxic chemicals with only a few phone calls or meetings. Sometimes it takes a more concerted effort, but the point is to not give up. It can be done, has been done, and you can do it.

Here are just a few steps to take and ways that moms have reported to us that worked.

1. Find out who makes the decisions.

2. Be friendly and get to know them—they are on your side!

3. Ask what chemicals they spray (do not assume), and when. Get names of the chemicals and the dates in writing.

4. Gather some brochures, studies, and a few friends.

5. Ask for a meeting with the decision maker in person or speak during open comments at your city council meeting.

6. Acknowledge them for all the work they do to care for and keep your city or school district safe. Let them see how they can be the town's heroes!

7. Present the information about why they need to stop spraying in a gracious, professional, and calm manner.

8. Offer solutions such as steam, mulch, and others as found on www.momsacrossamerica.com/toxin_free_town_campaign.

9. Ask if they will review your information and consider not spraying.

10. Follow up with them and/or your city council or board and be grateful for progress and their time. This may mean you'll have to speak at a city council or school board meeting, or it may not. Sometimes phone calls or petitions work, too.

11. Celebrate your success far and wide to inspire others!

People in Politics

The National Museum of the American Indian in Washington, DC, has a display of a beautifully feathered headdress. Underneath it is a tiny plaque that I just so happened to read when I visited the museum with my mother after marching in a Washington, DC, Fourth of July parade in 2014. It states, "The fifty chiefs of the Haudenosaunee grand council continue to be chosen by clan mothers, who also maintain the power to remove leaders based on lack of performance." Why is this? This is because the Haudenosaunee (also known as the Iroquois) community trusts that a mother's commitment is in alignment with the community's best interest.

By empowering the mothers to reclaim their power, to hold leaders to account, and be the people in power, we will transform the food industry. The mothers who buy 85 percent of the food, who are the backbones of our families, schools, churches, and communities can not only vote politicians in or out of office, we can *be* the people in office—and whether we are in office or not, we can ban GMOs and glyphosate from our tables, towns, and homes, right now.

In fall of 2016 I was honored to be hosted by Beth Savitt and the Shaka Movement to speak in Maui and experience the UNSTOPPABLE love or "Aloha" from the residents of Hawai'i for their community, earth, water, and families. Although they are ground zero for GMO open field test plots—and, in some areas of the island of Maui over sixty chemicals have been documented as sprayed up to nineteen times a day—they continue to have faith that they can make a difference and protect their community. Although the bills that they fought for and won fairly were later struck down by judges that sided with the chemical companies, the activists still have faith that their voices make a difference. Although hundreds of farm workers who are neighbors to the open GMO test plots sprayed with chemicals and children who live and play in the wake of plumes of toxic smoke from sugar fields that are burned after being sprayed with glyphosate have experienced severe harm, they have faith that their actions make a difference. Why? Because they do.

Despite enormous setbacks, every person who learns about the toxins and takes a step toward eliminating them makes a difference for their community, as does every person who stands up to corporate corruption, grows or buys organic, speaks at their city council, or runs for council. As I stood before the awe-inspiring group of activists and citizens, who marched in groups of three thousand or more before mainland Americans began to march, I said to them, "My husband believes that it is time to stop appealing to the people in power and *be* the people in power. That means many of you will need to run for office. Be the ones in power on your island—you have an opportunity to take back your community!"

Later that year in social media posts, I recognized the lovely faces of five people that I had seen in that audience who decided to run for city council. Joy filled my heart, and I knew that whether they won or not, they would continue to make great strides in Hawai'i. Not because of the laws, but because of their Aloha, or love, peace, and compassion for their people and land. Case in point, in May, 2018 Hawai'i became the first state to ban chlorpyrifos, a known neurotoxin. Something tells me that the people the activists recently elected into office had something to do with this. May we all follow their lead!

Contacting elected officials can also make a difference. Representative Ted Lieu of California listened to his constituent, scientist Stephen Frantz, and arranged for a congressional briefing on glyphosate herbicides in Washington, DC. It was a dream come true for Moms Across America. An experienced activist told me that congress never takes action on activists' behalf and that a glyphosate briefing was just "not going to happen." But one citizen who would not consider himself an activist (and perhaps did not "know better") asked his congressman to do the right thing, and he did. As a representative of mothers struggling with sick children, I was honored to be on the congressional glyphosate briefing panel with esteemed scientists. I was thrilled that the room was packed with congressional staffers. Afterward, we met with the EPA and presented our case. This time, inspired by communication with Séralini, the French molecular biologist, I asked the pesticide review board staff, "Do you have any long-term animal studies with blood analysis on the final formulation of Roundup?"

They said, "Which one? There are hundreds . . ."

I said, "Any."

They said, "No, not that we are aware of . . ."

"Then how can you claim that it is safe?" I was furious.

The director ended the meeting.

Since then, perhaps due to political pressure, the National Toxicology Program has agreed to assess the safety of the final formulations. The EPA will consider their findings in their review, which they said would be complete in 2015, then 2016 . . . 2017 . . . and now . . . 2018. The results, if the study is allowed to continue, could make or break their decision to reapprove glyphosate for another fifteen years. If it is halted, we have even more evidence that local action is crucial to protect our communities.

Mothers Across the World

After a food safety conference in Beijing, with thirty experts from fifteen countries around the world, I had the privilege of having Dr. Vandana Shiva, a world-renowned speaker, author, and environmental leader, sit with me during a three-hour bus ride to and from the Great Wall. She was generous with her insights, advice, and support. She suggested that we create a Mothers Across the World website to link mothers and expand our cause. So we did. Mothers Across Canada, Moms Across Ireland, and Mothers Across Africa were created—and then Mothers Across Japan. Although it is still in its infancy stage, the global platform has opened communication around the world. I have been invited to speak in China, Australia, New Zealand, Switzerland, Japan, and France. Regardless of where I am speaking, I see almost the same number of hands go up when I ask how many people have family members with health issues. It is heartbreaking and also highly motivating.

Other countries have done a far better job than Americans have at restricting GMOs and glyphosate. After our finding of glyphosate in breast milk in 2014, European countries such as Germany and France discontinued the practice of spraying glyphosate as a drying agent on crops. Sri Lanka has outright banned glyphosate herbicides after twenty thousand people, mostly young men who farmed with glyphosate herbicides, died of liver or kidney damage. Several thousand of these Sri Lankan citizens were women or children who never came in contact with glyphosate herbicides in the field. They did hug their husbands or fathers and consumed glyphosate in the water. The countries of Sri Lanka, El Salvador, Saudi Arabia, Kuwait, the United Arab Emirates, Qatar, Bahrain, and Oman have banned glyphosate. Malta, the Netherlands, and Argentina are in the process of banning glyphosate. The entire European Union, all twenty-eight countries, has refused to renew the license of glyphosate for fifteen years as the chemical companies expected. A controversial, last-minute change of heart (which went against Chancellor Merkel's wishes) by the minister of food and agriculture in Germany allowed a five-year renewal of glyphosate to pass in the EU, but France and Germany have since declared that they will ban glyphosate herbicides within three years, and the EU is expected to also make significant restrictions. Countries like Belgium and Austria have already banned glyphosate. No matter what, Roundup is on its way out in Europe. New Zealand, the United Kingdom, France, and Asia all have regions that have discontinued the use of glyphosate herbicides. Dozens of school districts, homeowner's associations, universities, and cities have begun to phase out the use of this harmful herbicide—and many other toxins, as well. Around the world, I have seen firsthand the urgency that citizens feel to rid their communities of toxic chemicals. I believe we have begun the *end* of the chemical era.

Speaking in other countries can be very overwhelming, and I am concerned about what I can say to help people. I am not an expert scientist or doctor. I am, however, an expert mom of my children, just as you are of your children or yourself. I am, however, an expert on being the mother of my children. As I step onto the stage in any country, I am determined that every person in the audience feels like they are also the expert on their own health and their family's health. The sight of the crowd in any country can be overwhelming because I can see the scope of the problem. Our food supply is a global issue; therefore, the health impact of food is global. It has been very daunting to have groups of mothers come up to me after my talks in China, Japan, and New Zealand and share horrifying stories of everything from rashes and near-death experiences from food allergies to cancer and severe autoimmune issues. These mothers are desperate and tired, but they are by no means giving up.

They have also been extremely grateful that I shared the testimonials of moms in America that were seeing improvements in their children's health. They are so relieved that so many had found solutions and are taking action. In China, a Buddhist farmer approached me, held both my hands, looked me earnestly in the eyes and said, "On behalf of one billion people and the mothers of China, I thank you." Tears welled up in my eyes. I knew it was not just me that she was grateful for, but all the mothers who had worked hard to find answers, who shared the truth, risked being ostracized, and spoke up to officials. I wished they could all have been with me to experience her gratitude.

In the spring of 2015 in Australia and New Zealand, hosted by MADGE (Mothers are Demystifying Genetic Engineering or Mothers Advocating Deliciously Good Eating) and GMO Free New Zealand, I met droves of mothers from the Weston A. Price Foundation who were more educated about toxins and health than most doctors. Their ability to study the functions of the human body and the interactions of certain vitamins and minerals in conjunction with foods was astounding. Mothers all around the world who reject GMOs are not anti-science—they are very much pro-science. In fact, they have learned more about the science than most doctors or food manufacturers have. They reject GMOs because they are reading and understanding more scientific studies than ever before.

October 2016 brought the Monsanto Tribunal at The Hague. Members of Navdanya, the Organic Consumers Association, Forum Civique Européen, Pesticide Action Network, and more organized a rousing People's Assembly held at the same time as the tribunal. I was deeply disturbed but grateful that the first two people to testify in the tribunal were mothers. They both had been exposed to glyphosate while pregnant and they both had babies who had birth defects and were undergoing dozens of surgeries. When I spoke later in the People's Assembly workshop on pesticides, I could see the impact on the faces in the audience when I described the harm that was happening to US children. There was no longer any debate in any of the attendees' minds that glyphosate herbicides, GMO farming, and the entire chemical farming system was poisoning us and killing off life on our planet.

In Japan in April 2017, on a ten-day speaking tour, I was moved when hundreds of enthusiastic mothers took a group photo with me at a GMO awareness conference. At this conference, not only did they share scientific facts about natural farming technology, seed sharing projects, and methods to raise awareness, but they also shared dancing, music, skits, and laughter. I have never seen such a joyous group of activists. I am sure that despite the enormous challenges before them, they will continue to make progress in protecting their children.

I saw evidence of many incredible community efforts in Japan. My host, the Green Co-Op Union of Japan, gave me a tour of the projects created by their co-op members. I visited a homeless shelter, fabric recycling center, nursery school, solar center, and Green Co-Op store in a devoted member's own home. All the projects were created by members of the co-op who buy their food directly from the food producers rather than from a grocery store. I was reminded of the rallying our moms did for the issue of clean water at Standing Rock. The health and safety issues of another community suddenly become your issues when you are connected to a caring group. This is how we become stronger—by simply being connected to community and taking action on behalf of all. These members saw needs in the community, such as healthy food for a school or a homeless shelter for instance, and they approached the co-op board members for support. The board, which consists entirely of mothers, considers the proposals and votes whether to support the projects. Their work is a wonderful example of how the community can begin by gathering around food but end up changing the very structure of a society.

Alter Trade Japan, a food distributor based in Tokyo, connected me with moms in the Philippines via a group Skype call. They shared about the pesticide use in nearby farms, and the health impact on their community, including the birth defects in babies of the farm workers. I learned that, according to Autism Speaks of the Philippines, at least one million, or *one out of every thirty-three,* children in the Philippines was diagnosed with autism in 2014. The rates of autism and developmental dysfunctions in Japan and South Korea were two to three times higher than the USA, which at the time—spring

2017—we knew to be one in sixty-eight children. I was stunned. I thought for sure their health was better than Americans'. Although we still don't know why this is happening, because no studies have been done comparing the impact of toxins in vaccines, pesticides in food, or the combination, we suspect that the major contributing factor is that Asians eat far more soy than we do, 99 percent of which is GMO from America. They also import the bulk of their food from other countries that use GMO and pesticide sprayed ingredients and are impacted by the toxins in agriculture, vaccines, and nuclear waste. I was thrilled to learn in November 2017 that the Philippine government had declared an outright, complete ban on GMOs. This bold step is sure to go a long way in reversing health issues.

> We can choose to create a future of health and freedom together, by sharing with one person at a time how we can opt out of GMO toxic chemical farming and choose organic farming instead.

In December 2017, new data emerged from the National Health Information Survey (NHIS), showing that one in thirty-three US children, and one out of twenty-eight boys, has been diagnosed on the autism spectrum.

Around the world, mothers are leading the way in grocery stores, doctors' offices, and our legislator's halls to protect their families' health. We see the impact immediately in our children's health from GMOs and toxins. We will do what it takes to protect them. As they say in Hawai'i, "We protect what we love."

Mothers Across the World has the potential to support an uprising of mothers who will stop the poisoning of generations. We have the ability to share the truth, stop the corruption, and change the world.

Dealing with Overwhelming News

When I first started Moms Across America, we were lucky if there was one article a week about GMOs. There was no media on glyphosate. None. Today, my Google alert lists dozens of articles every day that mention GMOs, Monsanto, or glyphosate—and it can be overwhelming to take it all in. I understand why some people turn off Facebook and don't forward emails for another petition. It's a lot. I get it.

The volume of news articles is, however, a testament to the great work so many activists and nonprofits are doing to raise awareness about the issue.

It is exciting that, because of the attention on this issue, new information is being discovered every day that can positively affect our health. New studies on the microbiome are fascinating. New studies on pesticides are crucial.

Here is how I handle all this information: I see it as an act of service to sort through the articles for the many people who do not want to, or do not have the time to, do so. I invite you to see it the same way. You may not be able to get out and pass out flyers for a few hours on the weekend, but you can definitely post an article or email a few hundred people in five minutes. You may not be the head of a nonprofit dedicated to raising awareness about these issues, but you are a leader for health in your family. You are looked up to by women in your circles or by people in your community because you bring organic snacks or manage to get your kid to eat something green. That does not go unnoticed—trust me.

By sharing information, you may become known as "the organic lady" or the "weird GMO guy." That's awesome. You have taken a stand for something. Embrace having taken that stand. Set a Google alert for the words GMO, glyphosate, and genetic engineering, which will alert you to national and international news on the subjects. Sign up for the Moms Across America newsletter. Sign up for the Organic Consumers Association or Sustainable Pulse newsletters. Be the one to scan the news. It takes less than five or ten minutes. Find one or two important articles and every day, or at least once a week, be the one to email out to your entire list or post the links to important, credible articles. You will become a resource for your community and a reliable source of the truth—and you don't even have to write a blog.

CHAPTER EIGHT
STEPPING INTO LEADERSHIP

"You must do the thing you think you cannot do."
—ELEANOR ROOSEVELT

NOVEMBER 2, 2012: it's election night, and I am sitting on a metal chair in an enclosed patio with a group of at least sixty other anxious people. More than who would be elected president, my family and I—and everyone else there—are on the edge of our seats to find out if Proposition 37, the California GMO labeling ballot initiative, has passed. Our fiery, redheaded leader Paula is at the front of the room and she is graciously acknowledging everyone's contribution. She has several people stand and share what they did and for how long. It is a wonderful space of acknowledgment, contribution, and gratitude.

I think about my part in the campaign, which was to pass out flyers at the farmer's market on Fridays as I shopped. It occurs to me that my role in the campaign had been very . . . convenient. Suddenly I realize that Paula is in the front of the room, and I am in the back of the room. I wonder to myself—why? I realize I had not taken on a role of leadership. I had only helped out. Nothing wrong with that—I did what I thought was best at the time. In my mind, I had separated the two, "leader" and "helper," and made them different. I thought being a leader required more responsibility and was therefore scary. I might mess up. To be a helper meant less responsibility and was, therefore, less scary. However, as Paula asked helper volunteers like me to stand up, I saw the helpers as leaders in their own way—they are leaders for their town. By acknowledging the contribution even the helpers made, and seeing we helpers as leaders too—the scariness began to melt. I saw I, too, was a leader. I felt good about what I had done, but I also began to wonder—what if I had taken on *more* leadership? I saw that if my actions would have been different—who knows what might have happened? Would my town have voted in favor? Possibly . . . and what about in the future? What if I took on that I am the one to transform the food industry? I began to see leadership as an opportunity.

As the evening progressed on election night, we got word that the labeling initiative had lost by a narrow margin. I walked out into the dark parking lot and found myself release months of anticipation that had just been dashed by tremendous disappointment. A dam burst, and I sobbed in the shadows. My chest heaved, and I gulped air, unashamed of crying in public. Kathleen, a peppy blonde, came up to me and said, "This is just the beginning. We are going to fight this!" I was so surprised by her determination. I clasped her hands and thanked her. Later she went on to help me with Moms Across America in the early months. Her hope and kindness will never be forgotten.

However, in the car that night, I continued to cry. I just could not believe that we had lost. Then my nine-year-old son Ben said quietly from the darkness, "Well you know Mom . . . even Star Wars took six episodes." Joy bubbled up and laughter flew out of my mouth, releasing my heart from the clench of sadness. My son's perspective delighted me. "Yes, you are right Ben—and they had Yoda." We laughed again. I realized maybe it was simply time for a new episode. Maybe this time I would take on leadership. My heart filled with love for my son. His wisdom dissolved my disappointment in the world. His clarity inspired me—and continues to inspire me daily.

I breathed in a deep, cleansing breath of air, and replenished my faith in life. Yes, it would take time. So many people still did not know about GMOs and the health risks they posed. I decided that I would be the one to transform the food industry. Not all by myself, but I would not wait for someone else to do something. I would take action now.

The following day, I obsessed over what I could or should have done differently, and what I could do next. Already frustrated, I spoke to my children's former school principal about his reaction to the movie I had lent him, *Genetic Roulette*. He said that he didn't believe that Monsanto was really that bad. My frustration faded as I began to boil with anger. The head of the PTA approached me that day as well. She asked me to change the Facebook page I had started for the school's parents to connect, to take off the words PTA, because I was posting about GMOs too much—and that was not a PTA issue. School lunch food was not a PTA issue? The next morning, I was still struggling and found myself once again crying—this time to my husband.

He said, "Zen, you are stressing about, and focused on, this one small school across the street. And they really can't do anything about the food supply. It's the system. You are playing too small a game. This is national. You need to play a bigger game."

> Is there a reason why you don't see yourself as a leader? What's holding you back?

He made me wonder . . . if I played a bigger game and took on a national focus . . . what could happen? He reminded me of a moment at Landmark, the personal development program, when a coach named Carlos Lopez said to me, "Zen, I request you take the lid off your leadership."

I said, "What do you mean? I am a Boy Scout den leader, I volunteer in the classroom every week, I am involved with the PTA, help the kids with their homework and getting to sports, and I volunteer to train public speaker leaders at Landmark seminar sessions. What more do you want from me?"

He smiled and said softly, "You think there is only so much you can do."

"Well, *yes*!" I said incredulously. "There really *is* only so much I can do!"

He held my gaze unflinchingly. "That's your lid," he said. "What if you took that lid off your leadership? What could be possible?"

I suddenly saw it. I saw my lid called "there is only so much I can do"—the lid I was not even aware I had before. It was just my perceived reality. I saw that I was constrained by that lid. It was my own point of view that was limiting me. I saw what he meant. If I stopped being limited by thinking, "There is only so much I can do," then all kinds of things could be possible. I could be the president or an astronaut or whatever . . . not that I wanted to be, but I saw what he meant.

My husband gave me the gift of thinking bigger—thinking national. Carlos, taking a few moments of his time, helped me see my lid and take it off. I *took on* being the one. I took on ownership, and leadership. I embraced the possibilities.

Be the Power. Go for What You *Really* Want. Now.

"Success is most often achieved by those who don't know that failure is inevitable."
—COCO CHANEL

Before Moms Across America, I was a fashion designer, working in New York, Montreal, Hong Kong, and Los Angeles for seven years. I learned how to design, do pattern making, and market products all together in a fast-paced industry. I stopped working to raise our children. When I had our first baby, I became concerned about toxins in body care products. I had health issues related to a lack of sleep, so I designed, made patterns for, and produced a collection of natural lavender wellness products. I called the line Zen's Purple Garden. A $465 billion Japanese cosmetic company that had trademarked the name Zen did not like that. They opposed my trademark and went so far as to tell me I could not even use the name, trademarked or not, for anything.

With coaching and a stance that "anything is possible," I got a lawyer and told him I wanted to negotiate with them to be able to use the name for whatever I wanted, without a trademark, I just wanted to keep doing what I was doing. He told me that based on his experience, he would advise against it, as I would inevitably fail. He said that it would take $20,000–$100,000 and two to five years, and that I would not get what I wanted.

It may have been naive, but I did not believe that his past experience had to be my future. I said, "Well I am coming from the belief that anything is possible. I have $2,000 and three months. Will you help me write a letter to them?"

He did. But he wanted me to compromise and not ask for lavender sprays because they were too close to their perfume. I refused. I would ask for everything I wanted. I would not censor my request or compromise.

The day of my self-imposed deadline, at 5:00 p.m., he called me and said, "I just got a fax from Japan, and they signed off on everything you wanted. I didn't think you had a shot in hell, but *you* did it."

I danced in the streets. I ran that company for as long as I wanted to—seven years. My kids got to see that you can create anything you set your mind to.

> Being naive about whether or not you can succeed can actually be a good thing! Who cares about the circumstances! Opposition too big? Do they have more money? Do they have more time and lawyers? Who cares! You are doing what is right. Go for it. You will achieve far more by creating what you want than by limiting yourself because you think something cannot happen.

I felt UNSTOPPABLE. But then, I found myself in the world of GMOs, an unchartered territory, and discovered I needed to learn this lesson again.

Shoot for the Moon

Norman Vincent Peale says, "Shoot for the moon. Even if you miss, you'll land among the stars." Too many people, even though they want the moon, don't shoot for the moon. Instead, they go for something more "grounded" and "reasonable" . . . and are disappointed when they get even less.

I believe this is why we lost GMO labeling. We asked for what was reasonable, for the least offensive, safest outcome: four simple words on the package: "Made With Genetic Engineering." We called only for identification—we did not ask for what we really wanted, which was a total ban. So, we got a compromise that was far less than reasonable . . . just a symbol, code, telephone number, or website. The words GMO will not need to appear anywhere on the package. That is not labeling. The Safe and Accurate Food Labeling Act of 2015 was passed to stop GMO labeling in Vermont, Maine, and Connecticut, and potentially in the forty-seven other states. The name is blatantly misleading, it does not make food safer. The cost argument put forth was also misleading. Putting four words on a label within two years' time would not have increased the price of the food. The government made a clear choice to pander to the chemical corporations.

When I asked leaders in the cause why we weren't fighting for a ban or at least a warning label during the GMO labeling initiative, the response I got surprised me. Apparently, I was naive. It just wouldn't work to take that strategy. The other activists knew for sure that we would not win a ban or warning label. So, I doubted myself and thought the leaders knew better because they knew "how the system works." I believed them. We all wanted to win *something*. We knew the odds against us were tremendous, but if we got labeling at least it would be a start. GMOs would be acknowledged. People could choose.

I see now what was missing from my own choice. I chose to support that "reasonable" movement rather than to fight for what I truly wanted. I didn't think my experience with Zen's Purple Garden applied to this case so I listened to others that I believed knew better than me. Right or wrong aside . . . lesson learned . . . again. No more. I want ALL GMOs and toxins *out* of our food, vaccines, homes, and environment. I want the freedom to choose what to feed my children, and what medical treatments they get. Period. To do that, we don't need to wait for our government to give us a ban on a silver platter. We definitely should not wait for the politicians to "see the light" through the piles of money that Monsanto, Dow, and DuPont have donated to them. We can ban GMOs ourselves through local community action. We all just need to trust ourselves, know the information, learn about the solutions, and know that what we are doing is best for current and future generations. As far as I was concerned, GMOs were already banned from my family's life, so my kids were as safe as I could have them be. My concern now was the bigger picture, not to ask for less for others than I would want for myself.

Robert Fritz says, "If you limit your choice only to what seems possible or reasonable, you disconnect yourself from what you truly want, and all that is left is a compromise." I hope that all leaders in all movements, whether the health freedom movement or other causes, will consider strategically that it will not work to compromise before you even ask for what you really want from the "powers that be." Don't give away your power.

What are the Possibilities?

Once I understood what was happening to the food supply I began to wonder—if actions I take would contribute to transforming the food industry, what would those actions look like? I asked myself—how could I reach as many people as possible in the shortest amount of time and educate them about GMOs?

A few minutes later, my first thought was *moms*. Moms are the ones with the purchasing power—we have a huge impact on the economy. Plus, people trust moms. They get that our only special interest is the well-being of our families. At first, I thought of marching on Washington, DC, but I knew the likelihood of moms flying across the country with strollers and babies and limited budgets was slim.

Next, and I don't know if I did it consciously or not, I put the tipping point concept used by Jeffrey Smith, together with Robyn O'Brien's phrase "Patriotism on a Plate." What if we could convince millions of Americans that it was in our nation's interest to reject GMOs and eliminate them from the food supply? Then, like a flower blooming, my mind went to the thought of local parades . . . Fourth of July parades. Millions of people plus a patriotic event! Moms everywhere could just join in! I was suddenly crystal clear. This would work. The port-a-potties, permits, and police would already be there, organized by someone else (easy!), it would be free or cheap to join in (affordable!), and the crowds could not ignore us (effective!). The cameras filming the parades might pick us up. We could join into events that had thousands of people lining the streets and reach millions across the country in a single day. It would be accessible, affordable, and appealing. With smiling faces, we could hand out flyers in person to our neighborhood! We could inform thousands who in turn would inform thousands of their friends . . . we could reach the tipping point in a family friendly, fun, and festive way!

I shared the idea with my husband, and he said, "Wow. That's huge. That's really, really, good." Then he looked concerned. He thought I often took on too much in my life. "You know that just because you have an idea doesn't mean you need to do it."

"Oh no," I said, sure as a clear blue sky. "I need to do this."

I was vibrating with a newfound energy. All my life I had had good ideas and was dismayed that I had never had a great idea. This time, though, I knew in my bones that it was a great idea—great as in, it could be highly effective. And yet, it was not a new idea. Thousands of groups join in Fourth of July parades every year—it just had not been encouraged and supported as a national activist outreach effort in our cause. I knew it would be a huge undertaking to have it be national and would take a lot of work. I would need to do things I had no idea how to do. I did not know how to make a website, or create a nationwide event, or support the marchers with banners and materials. I did not know how to fundraise large amounts of money or how to start a nonprofit.

In a Landmark class, the instructor told the crowd, "You are going to have to rearrange the molecules of your being to be the person you are creating."

He explained that when you have a big game—a big, hairy, audacious goal—you make a difference for others and transform an area of life that matters to you. The person you are when you create that possibility is not the same person you will need to be to fulfill that possibility—to make it come alive and be real in the world. You will need to rearrange the molecules of your being . . . essentially expand upon who you are, or reinvent yourself.

I got it. The person you are when you get a job is not the same person that is successful at that job a year or two later. You need to learn a lot, change, grow, give up old habits, create new ones, create new relationships and teams, and achieve your desired outcomes. You are a different person—a person who has rearranged the molecules of her being to be who you said you would be. That concept scared the wits out of me. But I wanted it.

You could change the world if you answer the following questions for yourself in earnest. (Just take your lid off first.)

How to Change Your World . . . How to Change *the* World

1. What is it that you want?
2. What problem do you want to solve?
3. How do you want the world/your life to be?
4. What is it that you are committed to?
5. What action can you start with?

I knew that I:

- Wanted to get rid of GMOs and toxic chemicals from our food.

- Wanted to solve the problem of sick kids/families and have them be well.

- Wanted a world where food and the environment were safe for our children.

- Was and am committed to health and freedom.

- Saw that I could take action—inviting people to join in Fourth of July parades—to educate as many people as possible in the shortest amount of time and make a difference in transforming both the food industry and the world.

The idea of creating a nationwide movement to join into Fourth of July parades was daunting. None of that mattered when I envisioned how beautiful it would be . . . old friends and new friends walking together in their local parade, smiling, waving, and raising awareness in a fun way. I envisioned community members connecting and listening to each other, not feeling alone anymore, and supporting others to find out how to heal themselves through food. Neighborhood spectators sitting on the sidewalks, eating chips and drinking soda, would nudge each other and say, "What's a GMO?" By getting curious, they might learn about a new pathway to health—possibly altering their family and generations to come. It would be so life changing for so many! No matter what I had to learn or do, I knew it would be worthwhile.

> When considering making a difference, ask yourself:
>
> 1. How could I make the largest impact in the shortest amount of time?
>
> 2. What big event, national holiday, gathering, or deadline is coming up?
>
> 3. What would work for others?
>
> 4. Is it affordable, easy to join, easily replicable, and fun?
>
> 5. How can I make this event available to thousands to join?
>
> This is an inquiry that, if done in any area of your life, for any cause, could literally transform the world. Your answers to these questions, if they come from love and being present to your commitment, will alter the future of the planet.

Yeah, But...

Consider that as soon as you have an idea, as excited as you will be about it, you will also immediately have all the reasons why you should *not* do it. The committee in your head will say, *Yeah, but...*

- I don't know how.

- I am too tired.

- I am too busy.

- I don't have enough money.

- I am not good at asking people for help.

- I am not an expert in this area—not credible enough.

I get it. These thoughts and more will inevitably show up.
I am now going to say two words that will eliminate all their power.
So what?
Really—*so what?*
So you don't know, are tired, or don't have enough money? So what? You may take this as a callous statement. I understand. Of course, you need to take care of your well-being and be responsible for your obligations and finances. No one is asking you not to be. But should you make a decision based on those concerns? What is more important to you—those thoughts in your head, or what you are committed to?

I would venture to say that if you knew you could bring this idea to life, empower millions, *and* not have your obligations neglected, you would do it. You can. Will there be difficult choices to make? Yes. Will there be big requests that you will need to make to obtain partnership for your other obligations at home, work, and social life? Yes. Will there be breakdowns and failures? Yes. So what? No biggie. You got this. You have community. You are never alone!

Difficult choices, asking for help, giving up control to others, delegating responsibility, taking on something that you don't know whether it will be a success or not, suffering breakdowns, and having failures all mean something wonderful. You are *up to something big*.

Bigger than yourself, bigger than your concerns. Doing that big thing is in alignment with our commitment—and that is what makes life full and rich and good. When you are clear about what you are committed to, everything else comes into focus and makes sense.

The "buts" usually come from fear of failure, of wanting to prevent a breakdown, or of wanting to avoid looking bad. Landmark leader Mark Spirtos told me, "Stop being afraid of getting it right. Start looking for ways to have breakdowns—which lead to breakthroughs. If you are not having breakdowns, that means you are not up to anything big. Look to cause breakdowns worthy of your life!"

I reminded myself every time a breakdown seemed to be happening . . . when volunteers who said they would help with planning the parades didn't show up, or a store wouldn't donate to support us . . . that there was a breakthrough around the corner. This is a major source of power for being UNSTOPPABLE . . . not being afraid of breakdowns, but actually embracing them as access to breakthroughs.

We are all going to have problems and breakdowns . . . do we want these breakdowns to be small ones such as missing a favorite TV show because of a flat tire on the way home to watch it? Or big ones like solving the issue that matters to you, such as feeding five hundred people for a fundraiser for children with cancer; eliminating joblessness in your town, ensuring clean water or air, or helping build better schools? When we have and expect breakdowns, we can also expect and create big breakthroughs that enable us to do great things.

> **How to be Fearless in the Face of Failure**
>
> What would you do if you couldn't fail?
>
> 1. Focus on what you are committed to.
>
> 2. MAKE YOUR GOAL BIG.
>
> 3. Stay focused even when things are not working.
>
> 4. Take action no matter what.

The lack of integrity in the food system is a breakdown, but the food movement is a breakthrough. We are coming together in beautiful and courageous ways . . . over 170 groups of moms and supporters joined in parades and reached hundreds of thousands of people locally and millions nationally with our GMO info flyers and banners in just a few months after the inception of Moms Across America.

The First Parade

"Wide awake I can make my most fantastic dreams come true."
—LORENZ HART

When you imagine something for months and then the moment is finally upon you, life feels surreal because it is inevitably not exactly as you had imagined. Sometimes it is bigger, brighter, and even more beautiful. The Moms Across America march in Fourth of July parades was like that for me. I couldn't believe it was happening—and yet, it felt exactly right.

It was a clear, sunny day in Connecticut. It was hot but not scorching and there was a slight breeze now and then—just enough to bring a sigh of relief. We gathered in the Stop & Shop parking lot in the charming and affluent town of Madison. Groups of cheerleaders, firefighters, men driving tiny cars, floats, and trucks gathered in colorful groups around us. I was beaming with excitement and felt more alive than I had felt in months. Leafy, green trees lined the streets, which were packed with parade spectators in their beach chairs.

My family was with me, all decked out in their GMO? We're NOT Buying It! and LABEL GMOs NOW! Because We Said So! T-shirts, holding signs we had made.

Around 10:00 a.m., it was our turn to start moving and join in the parade. Karen, the local leader, and I each grabbed our sons and the banner and began to walk. I couldn't believe we were in a parade and that this was happening all across the country! I thought of Laurie Olson in Washington who had helped to support fourteen parades happening in her state, the Florida leaders who had twelve across their state, Kathleen, John, and a large group who were in a parade at Huntington Beach, California, which had two hundred thousand attendees, and over 170 other groups across the country—reaching millions that day. How amazing! As we turned the corner onto the main parade route, families that were all looking at us lined both sides. As we marched down the street, our group spread out to reach only a few feet from either side. We waved, smiled, and chanted for GMO labeling as thousands clapped for us and waved back. They were asking us and each other,

"What is a GMO?" It was exhilarating! My heart buzzed with joy! Mission accomplished!

My sister, Chi, and my brother-in-law, Tim, pushed a bike trailer with both my youngest son, Bronson, and their daughter, Kaia, in it. My brother, Tao, pushed a shopping cart with a GMO-Free Shopper sign on it while my middle son, Bodee, sat in the cart and peered at the crowd. My sister-in-law Amy, though not a mom, but a caregiver of the highest sort, smiled while waving a plate decorated with the image of the US flag. My eldest son, Ben, marched proudly beside me along with about a dozen Connecticut residents.

My mother, Mavis, who was seventy-two years old, beamed with joy and held the sign she had made, while she chatted with the other participants. A family from Massachusetts came to march with us, all wearing matching black Non-GMO T-shirts. They ran up and down the crowds on the sides of the streets, passing out thousands of flyers. Periodically we all sang the first two verses of a song I wrote with farmer Howard Vlieger, "This Land We Want GMO Free" to the tune of "This Land Is Your Land, This Land is My Land." We had a ball! To have met so many dedicated, generous people and feel instantly connected with them, was such a blessing.

At one point during the parade, I switched places with one of the kids who was passing out flyers and let him hold the banner. It was so fun to pass out our brochures, look people in the eye and say, "Thank you for finding out more about GMOs!" or "We hope your family will be healthy and happy!" or "Do you know about GMOs? This will change your life!" When we made eye contact, I felt like I really was making a difference in their lives—I was showing them a new pathway to health. They might not choose to take that path, but at least they now knew they had options. I gave flyers to grandmas who were cheering for us and to grumpy grandpas who at first wanted to wave me away but then gave me a shrug and a smile. I gave flyers to children to pass back to their parents and to teens who actually thanked me. I got to experience human beings as grateful, willing, and open.

I was reminded of the time when my sons handed out Moms Across America flyers at a local Irvine Global Village Festival and as I watched them approach people, the voice in my head said silently to the passersby, "Please take a flyer from them!" I so wanted my sons to feel successful in making a difference for others and to experience other people as kind and willing. A beautiful elderly lady stopped and looked at my sons, saying, "What do you have there, Sweetie?" She gave them her full attention and they perked up, stepped forward, and clearly felt important.

I don't know if many are present to this, but when someone wants to give you something, and you accept it, you are doing them a great service. When people took the time to accept the flyers and say thank you to my sons even though they did not know what the flyer was about, my sons lit up, stood taller, came back empty-handed and full of confidence and happiness. I am grateful to that kind lady and all those generous people for contributing to my sons' development. I felt the same way at the parade—grateful to every person who willingly accepted a flyer. You are being generous when you say yes, and I thank everyone who has ever accepted one of our flyers from our supporters across America. You have made a difference in our lives, too. Thank you.

Marching merrily in the raucous parade, we rounded a corner and were announced from the judging booth. "Next up, we have Moms Across America, a National Coalition of UNSTOPPABLE Moms," there was cheering, "whose motto is 'Empowered Moms, Healthy Kids.' They are marching for healthy food, GMO labeling, and the right to know what is in our food. Let's hear it for the moms!"

I felt love and light radiating through me. It was a moment I will never forget. Moms all across the country were experiencing this—being cheered on for taking a stand for the health of their children and country. If they felt even 10 percent as good as I did, it was all worth it!

The three miles was a long way to walk under the hot sun. When one of the trucks in front of us misted water, the kids and I ran up and got wet enough to cool ourselves down a few degrees. I thought of all the people marching down south in even hotter weather and silently thanked them for their commitment.

Eventually, there were less and less people on the sides of the streets and we turned off the main road to a smaller road heading toward the park. We saw the band of pipers peeling off layers of wool uniforms and taking off hats and I thanked God we only had organic cotton T-shirts as our uniforms.

We stopped in a group and, although it felt anticlimactic, I thanked everyone for their participation and acknowledged Karen again for her leadership in organizing the event. We all clapped and commented about how great it had been. "There were so many people cheering! They know about GMOs! They were really glad to see us! What a surprise!" We felt less alone—like we were surrounded by supportive community. I was in love with the people of America.

It was sad to see people disperse right away to get out of the heat, but I was glad when the family from Massachusetts stayed at the park with us while we all ate a picnic lunch in the cool, soothing shade. We talked about the movement, the tragedies, and the triumphs. We might differ on politics or religion, but we all ate, we all cared about our health, and—unfortunately—we all loved someone who was sick. We would do anything for them and for our common future. We would travel through states, march in ninety-degree heat, pass out flyers to strangers, and spend our time and money without expectation of compensation. It was a beautiful, creative, and courageous moment.

We estimated that with only ten thousand people at each of the 170 parades (some had five thousand, some had fifty thousand and some had as many as two hundred thousand), we reached more than a million and a half people in person and millions more through the televised parades and social media in a single day. We did this. Every mom and supporter who said, "Okay, I will gather some friends and join in a parade to let my whole town know about GMOs," did this. Moms and families, without millions of dollars of advertising, without the promise of being elected to office, and without fame or fortune, did this.

I know that some people might feel Moms Across America toots our own horn a little too much, but we are going to keep on tooting, because our moms deserve it. Moms are the unsung heroes of every culture. We are the backbone of our churches, schools, sports clubs, and scout groups. We organize the social gatherings, the family events, and many of the community events. We get our Moms Across America name and logo out as much as possible, because we want moms to be proud of what we are accomplishing together, to be boldly outspoken, fully acknowledged, and inspired to be brave and to try something new. We amplify the voice of the moms because for too long we have been ignored. And what we have to say is crucial if our human race is going to not only survive, but also thrive. We celebrate the successes of moms, because their love and strength in our communities could turn our country around to go in the right direction. The parades gave us the impetus to begin.

The parades were new for our movement at the time. I didn't ever remember seeing an activist group in a Fourth of July parade. I hope after our events and the release of this book, we will see many other groups focusing on different issues join in the parades—fracking, climate change, health choice, money in politics—these causes could all reach so many people in Fourth of July parades.

> *When we first started, one out of fifty people knew about GMOs. Now, after we have been marching in parades, and with the support of Moms Across America, one out of fifty people I meet does not know about GMOs. I am proud to be a part of that shift.*
> —Laurie Olson, MAA board president

A Note to Introverts Like Me

I just shared about marching in a parade in front of thousands of people. That might scare the pants off some people—particularly introverts. I get it. I invite you to consider that we need everyone to create the world we want—everyone . . . and introverts have a crucial role to play.

I am, by nature, what most people would call an introvert. I like to be alone. I am intimidated by social situations and can often appear very serious, unapproachable, aloof, or socially awkward. I have, in the past, shied away from groups and that would stop me from getting involved with political groups or activism. I can see now that my desire to shy away from situations that interest me but scare me is an instinctual reaction to stay comfortable. It's automatic.

> Whether you consider yourself an introvert, an extrovert, or something in between, I encourage you to relish in the gifts that you bring to the table—and to also honor other people, no matter what their styles.

Automatic only works for behaviors like brushing my teeth or putting my foot on the brake for a red light. Automatic, default behavior does not work for rich, loving relationships, listening to and empowering others, or creating change in the world. This is a very challenging concept for most people to apply to their lives. By recognizing that fears are automatic and could limit your actions, you can choose to create new actions not based on your automatic fears, but instead based on the future that you want to create—like one of health and freedom. What you are committed to—that future—is more important than automatic fears.

If you are interested in stepping outside your comfort zone and becoming a local leader, a speaker, or an organizer, do it. If that path isn't right for you or isn't right for you now—then take the path that *is* right for you. Take action anyway! We need all kinds of people to transform the food supply and health in America. We need people who consider themselves to be introverts who excel at details, design, and data. We need thoughtful, careful people to crunch numbers, plan events, and go through letters and speeches with a fine-tooth comb. And yes, we need speakers, rabble-rousers, and tambourine bangers, too. Do whatever moves you . . . do something.

CHAPTER NINE
SPEAKING TO FRIENDS, FAMILY, AND STRANGERS

"Faith is taking the first step even when you don't see the whole staircase."
—MARTIN LUTHER KING, JR.

I WAS AT a BBQ in the park at the end of our street in the spring of 2013. A neighbor had invited a few friends to get together and I got to chatting with one of the moms. She was concerned about her son's behavior. He was heavyset, loud, and difficult to communicate with at times. He did not respond to his mother or follow her directions. She was clearly frustrated. I asked her if she knew anything about GMOs, and she said no. I told her how they are a foreign protein in the majority of our foods and could possibly be irritating his stomach lining. I told her about the gut/brain connection, and the rats from the lifelong study that had tumors, sex hormone changes, and even birth defects and infertility. As her brow furrowed in concern, I stopped myself.

"Is this too much?" I asked. After all, it was just a BBQ and I didn't know her well.

"No!" she said staring straight into my eyes. "This is my kid you are talking about. You need to tell me these things. I *need* to know."

In that moment, I decided to trust myself and not hold back. Every mother, every parent, regardless of how inconvenient, wants to know what might be harming their child so they can stop it, or take precautions and prevent it from happening in the first place.

Every mother, *every* parent, wants to know, regardless of how expensive new action might be, what they can do to protect their child.

How to Talk about GMOs and Toxins

If your family and friends do not know, or believe what you tell them, about GMOs and toxins, this can be incredibly frustrating. I have been there. I know what it feels like to watch loved ones eat what you know to be poison and feel deeply saddened and frightened for them.

I offer you ways to create a foundation of open communication and five methods you can use to talk with your family or friends about GMOs. We all need to speak up for the sake of our entire community and future generations.

> When it comes down to it, nothing is too difficult to hear or do if it pertains to the health of our child. The truth frees us from enslavement to the status quo. It empowers us to a new course of action. It opens up possibilities.

Before you begin, just for a moment get present to the way you normally talk to your family about this topic or other topics that may seem controversial. Pick a single person to focus on. Your mother. Or sister. Or dad. How does the conversation usually go? What do you say, and then what do they say? How do you feel? Do you feel tense and defensive? Frustrated?

Consider for a moment that how we think a conversation is going to go has a lot to do with what will actually happen. We can create tension, frustration, or resentment in a conversation just by expecting it to go in a certain way. We often speak in a way that generates the anticipated outcome, even if that's not the outcome that we actually want.

For instance, if I expect my sister to be busy and act dismissive about a certain topic, when I address it with her I might say, "You are probably busy, but I want to talk to you about something." The way I present it sets her up to agree she is busy and then be dismissive. We often create the very thing we are trying to prevent.

We don't have to do this. Instead, we can come from a place of love—a place of no expectations, of curiosity, and of creation. For a moment, in your mind's eye, sweep away all those past conversations, whether they were about GMOs or other topics. Clear your mind. Start fresh. Ask yourself . . . what are you creating? What are you committed to in your relationship with this person? Love? Connection? Health? It may be many things—but for a number of us, it all comes down to love, empowerment, health, and freedom. Focus on one or two words. Whatever it is for you, can you see that creating a conversation from that commitment will be much more effective than coming from an expectation of tension, frustration, or misunderstanding. *you* are the *one* to create what you are committed to: love, health, empowerment, and freedom—or whatever else you want to create. You are the one. No matter what. And then be open to creating something new.

Because there are endless possibilities in communication, and there are many different types of people whose perspectives of what is valid or important differ, I invite you to read through the six different ways to communicate that I offer and then chose one to start. Be open to a multitude of outcomes, but also be willing to try it exactly the way I suggest. First, create a foundation of open communication.

Create a Foundation of Open Communication

1. Be Interested in What Matters to Her

First, ask yourself—does the person you are talking to feel like *she* matters to you? (Let's say, for the sake of this discussion, that this person is a woman—perhaps your mother or sister.) That you care about what *she* thinks or feels? Or does she think you just want to get her to do things *your* way? Or that you know better than she does, and you just want to convert her, so to speak? If so, you may need to apologize for your past behavior before you start a new a conversation.

Make sure to be *present, fully focused on her and her world*. Let's choose for this example, your sister. Ask your sister how she is, how her life is, what is happening with her. Listen. Do not interrupt and do not try to fix anything. Do not give advice—just get her. Really, really get her. This may feel uncomfortable—but that means you are trying something new. *Good.* Trying something new is good!

2. Get in Her Shoes

Does your sister feel heard, that you get where she is coming from, and that you are trying to understand what her life is like? You can have her feel that you understand her by really being present to what she is committed to, and in your communication, that will show in a certain way. For instance, if she says that she is trying as hard as she can, but she just can't figure out why her daughter Mia has a rash, you might try to *fix it* by saying, "Have you tried neem cream?" Or you could be in denial and *be nice* by saying, "You are doing the best you can—she'll be fine. It's just a rash."

Instead, *after* she is completely done sharing, caring about what she is committed to might sound something like, "This must be super frustrating for you. You know Sis, I really acknowledge your commitment to Mia's health. You have been trying different creams for three years now and you haven't given up. You're UNSTOPPABLE! Mia is so lucky to have you for a mom. She must know how much you love her—at least I do." Understand that, no matter what your sister's complaint, she is really coming from love . . . and a whole new conversation and a whole new relationship will unfold.

3. Understand That You Could Live with It If She Stayed Exactly the Same

People do not want to feel like something is wrong with them. There is nothing more loving than to really accept—and not just accept, but truly cherish—a person for exactly the way she is. Say something like, "Sis, you know that whether Mia's rash gets better or not, that you are an *awesome* mom. You know that, right?" When you say something like this, really mean it. Be present to the fact that if nothing ever changed, she would still be the loving mom she is, doing the best she can—and is perfect the way she is. Let her know that!

4. Ask If You Can Share Something You Have Learned

You will know that she really gets you and how much you love her, when she looks you in the eye and it is clear that she is truly touched. She might even be moved to tears. There is nothing more important than for you to get her completely and be present to how much you love her. Then, ask her, "Have you ever heard about GMOs?" If she says no—or even if she says yes—ask her if you can share with her something that you have recently learned that you think might be helpful. Ask for permission. If she says no, respect that and wait for another time. If she says yes, then share what you learned. Briefly. Simply. Gently. Speak authentically.

You may say something like, "I just learned that our food has changed. Chemical companies have invented genetically modified seeds that grow even though farmers spray toxic chemicals on them—and our FDA allows this. Those GM seeds are corn, soy, sugar, and lots of other different foods we feed our kids every day. I was really mad to learn that the chemicals do not wash off. The chemicals can cause rashes in kids, and the rash is the body's way of communicating that there is inflammation happening in the gut. The rash is a good thing! *There is nothing wrong with what you are doing.* It's the food. It's different. It's not the same as it was when you and I were kids. But what I have learned, and others are seeing, too, is that when they switched to organic, whole foods, their health issues improved, including rashes going away, preventing more serious disease, too."

Method One: Feel, Felt, Found

Adapted from a sales technique, Feel, Felt, Found is very effective in connecting with people respectfully and inviting them to see something new—in this case, the "something new" is that they *can* do something about their family's health.

After you share the basic concept of GMOs, be ready for the "buts" . . . the contradictory comment, or shutdown, or opposition. It's just human nature. No one wants to change. Do *not* take it personally.

Here is where Feel, Felt, Found comes in. For instance, if she says, "Really? You know . . . I heard something about genetic whatever and pesticides, from Aunt Annie, but I just can't afford it." (Or, "I don't have the time to shop/cook," or, "I can't find organic anywhere.") First, get her communication by looking her in the eye and saying, "I know how you **feel**." Then say, "I **felt** the same way." You might add a personal example, "When I saw that organic bread costs almost twice as much as my regular loaf, I freaked out."

Then you say, "But you know what I **found**? I found that when I didn't buy soda, I could easily afford organic bread. I felt better after I ate it, my stomach didn't hurt, and after about a week or two I didn't even miss the soda! I use organic lemons and stevia now for a sweet drink. The kids love it, and we all love the organic bread."

Or, you may use an example from another person. "But you know what I found? When I researched the benefits of eating organic food, I **found** several blogs by people whose kids had multiple allergies and rashes that went away just by going organic. They even still ate sweets now and then. The major change was just switching to organic!"

If she says she doesn't have enough time, you may say. "I know how you **feel**. I **felt** the same way. The kids have sports, I work late, and my husband travels a lot, and it is stressful. Cooking at home seems like it would just add to the stress . . . but you know what I found? I **found** that when I prepared a few meals and organic granola bars or muffins on Sunday while I watched an old movie, I was so much happier the rest of the week because that stress was gone!"

After One Example, Be Quiet

This is often the hardest part. If you keep talking, they will feel overwhelmed and shut down. Be quiet after you give one personal example of what you've found. *Stop talking.* This will feel very counterintuitive. You will want to open the floodgates and tell them one hundred reasons why they should change the way they are eating. You will want to give them articles and website links and point to all the words you have so carefully and thoughtfully taken the time to highlight. Don't do this. Trust me. Give them one example and then zip it! Or, as my mother would say, *enjoy the silence.*

Wait for Her to Ask You a Question

Just wait. It might feel awkward. You might have to pour a glass of water, pet your cat, or do whatever will keep you from talking. Do what you need to but remain available and present to the conversation. After a moment, maybe after recuperating from the surprise that you are not going to say anything more, lecture, or preach, your sister will most likely say something like, "Really? Can you show me that blog?" Or, "Where do you buy organic?" If she is interested and she asks, then she will be much more likely to make changes. Wait for *her* to show interest.

Give Her One Easy Step She Can Start With

Do *not* overwhelm her. Start with, "Sure I will email you that blog after dinner." Or, "I buy a lot of organic food from the farmer's market on Friday. Would you like to go with me this week?" *Then leave it at that.*

Follow-Up

A few days later, give her a call and check in, ask her how she is, listen to her, acknowledge her, and then ask if she had any trouble finding organic food. If she did have trouble, ask her if you can help by taking her shopping. Supporting her shopping could get her kick-started in a healthy direction.

Acknowledge Her

After she makes even one change, even if it's just switching to organic soda and chips, acknowledge the heck out of her. Be *so* happy. *Smile.* Hug her.

High-five her. Let her know you are really glad. Encourage everything that is going in the right direction. Do not make a big deal about the choices that are not organic. Most importantly, get present to how much you love her—there is nothing more important than that.

Method Two: Entertain Them

Most people love watching movies. Most people prefer to hear information from people who are *not* members of their family. If you have a family member who likes to watch movies, try entertaining him or her instead.

After everyone is fed, rested, and connected, look a loved one (for example, your Dad) in the eye and say, "Dad, will you watch this movie with me? Then, afterward, can we talk about it?" He might be begrudging, but usually our loved ones will say okay.

Then, after the movie, skip directly to feel, felt, found.

We have dozens of movies to choose from on our website. www.momsacrossamerica.com/movies_about_gmos

Method Three: Call in the Troops

Some people will only believe something if they can see it in black and white and it consists of references to or is a peer-reviewed, published, scientific study. They need to hear it from a doctor, scientist, or triple platinum expert in their field. So, give them that!

Go to www.momsacrossamerica.org/data and download the studies that look most relatable to that person. Men might be more interested in the studies about testes and sex hormone disruption. New mothers might be more interested in the study that shows goats produce less milk on GMO feed. Grandparents might be more interested in the studies that show epigenetic harm—that future generations can be impacted.

Gather between three and six scientific studies, highlight a few points, and bring them to your loved one. Give them to this person with a very short introduction. "I found these studies about GMOs and glyphosate, and I am curious to know what you think about them."

Do not say, "These studies *prove* what I have been saying for three years. Here—read them!" You would be lucky if your family member even glanced at them. Do not make it about you being right and them being wrong. Be curious about what *they* think.

If your family member prefers books:

- For law lovers, I suggest Steven Drucker's book *Altered Genes, Twisted Truth* or the nonprofit US Right to Know's Carey Gillam's book, *Whitewash*.

- If they value science, but probably won't read or understand scientific studies, give them the book *Poison Spring* by Evaggelos Vallianatos, a former twenty-nine-year employee of the EPA, or *Seeds of Destruction* by Jeffrey M. Smith.

- If they enjoy history, share the *War on Bugs* by Will Allen or *Foodopoly* by Wenonah Hauter of the nonprofit Food and Water Watch, or *Kiss the Ground* by Josh Tickell.

- Parents will enjoy *GMO-Free Child* by April Scott Keyes, *The Unhealthy Truth* by Robyn O'Brien, or *What's Making Our Children Sick?* by Dr. Michelle Perro.

- Cooks on a budget will enjoy the informative book *15 Minute Healthy, Organic Meals for Less than $10 a Day* by Susan Patterson.

Sometimes, *you* are one of the troops. You are the resident expert about GMOs for your family. So sometimes, you may offer to help them and really commit to supporting them in learning about GMOs and improving their health issues. If this is appropriate and welcome, carve out the time to guide them and shop with them. It's worth it.

Method Four: Come Bearing Solutions

Some people are open to bad news and want to know the worst. Other people are averse to hearing bad news. Telling them about the dangers of the food supply will make their faces cloud over and you will lose their attention. They may even avoid you.

Instead of loading them up with studies, having a deep conversation, or handing them a huge book on the volumes of science behind GMOs, take a different approach. Do an activity with them instead! Say, "I am having some ladies over to make sauerkraut [or kombucha, or kefir cheese] on Saturday, do you want to come?" Have *fun* with them making something healthy and delicious! While you are squishing the whey out of the cheese or pounding the juice out of the cabbage, you might casually mention, "I was so glad to find Donna Schwenk's website www.culturedfoodlife.com, because when I learned about GMOs and all the pesticides in the food, I was really overwhelmed. I thought, what am I supposed to feed my family? It felt like I would have to take a whole lot of stuff out of their diet that they love! So, when I found her site I realized I could first focus on adding the good stuff *into* their diet and see a lot of benefits. On the video on her site, Donna says her daughter recovered from eleven food allergies in just one year! She says that cultured (fermented) foods have up to one trillion good bacteria in a tablespoon and balance out the gut biome. That's easy! I can do that!"

Then let your friends ask questions if they want to, but don't talk about it for too long. In fact, you might say, "I am not the expert in this area, but I have a movie I have been wanting to watch about GMOs to learn more from the experts. I can show it next week if you want to come over and watch it with me." Then just enjoy them for the rest of the night. *Do not be overwhelming about this information!*

After watching the movie together, you could:

- Go grocery shopping with them and casually point out alternatives to what they usually buy.

- Show them how much money they can save by buying bulk and eating organic at home by crunching some numbers. Share the MAA blog "Does Organic Food Cost Too Much?"

- Cook organic meals together—maybe with organic wine—and just enjoy being together and eating delicious, safe food!

Which comes to our next method for talking about GMOs and toxins with your family . . .

Method Five: Don't Talk—Feed Them!
Some people really won't want to talk about GMOs and the food supply. They just don't believe what you say, don't think it's appropriate for a young'un to tell an elder how to eat, or really do think they are smarter than you in just about every way possible. It happens. It's okay.

Or maybe you have no idea what they think about GMOs, but you do know that *everyone* loves to eat delicious food! So . . . invite everyone over for a dinner party! Just because. Feed them 100 percent organic food—maybe vegan or vegetarian, if you choose—and don't tell them. After dessert, before they leave, put out a sign that says, "If you liked the way we eat, take one," next to a stack of our flyers about GMOs and "Why eat organic?" flyers. Laura, in Washington, DC, did this, and every flyer was gone at the end of the evening. She had not said one word about GMOs.

Another mom, Illana in Michigan, also held an organic dinner party and invited her guests to come back another time for a movie screening of *GMO OMG,* at her home. They watched the movie together and have unofficially formed an email thread support group. They share the names of stores that are selling new organic products, support each other with organic supplement suggestions, and get together once a month for a new movie screening. Once again—in that first gathering, she never once discussed GMOs or pesticides. She just enjoyed their company.

So, if there is anything that you take away from these five methods for talking to your family about GMOs, I hope you take away that getting present to how much you love your family member *is the most important thing.* When you get how much you love them, and when they get how much you love them, anything is possible.

Public Speaking

"Courage is resistance to fear, mastery of fear, not absence of fear."
—MARK TWAIN

I am sure many of us can think of a moment from our childhood—perhaps in school—when speaking up was suddenly seen as not a safe thing to do. In order to survive, we decided to stay silent. Suppressing our voices became our new normal.

There is a time however, when the status quo is no longer okay and most of us feel compelled to speak up. It could have been running for student council, making a toast for a wedding, speaking up at a Cub Scout meeting or church group, or giving a presentation at work. There is a time when we need to—whether we want to or not—speak up among our peers or stand up in front of a group of strangers. Making a difference with a large group of people about any cause requires someone willing to speak about the topic and rally others.

In polls, public speaking is rated the number one fear of all humankind. Death is number two. *That means people would rather die than speak in public.* When I found myself speaking in front of my high school student body and I said something inappropriate, everyone laughed at me, and I wanted to die. For me, the fear of public speaking is compounded by fears of messing up and being laughed at.

Creating a future of health and freedom for my children meant that I needed to get past those fears and not let them stop me from sharing the crucial information that I had learned. In my journey to become a public speaker, it has become one of my favorite things to do. The following are some ways to not only overcome fears, but also learn to love public speaking.

Practice

Public speaking takes practice. The nature of habit is what tells your fight-or-flight instinct that you have done this before, you survived, it's safe, and you can do it again. So, getting back on the horse really does work. I practice in front of the mirror, working on making eye contact and looking at my notes as little as necessary. If I can look at the person in the mirror with confidence, I can look at anyone. I am my own toughest critic.

Practice until you are comfortable with the words you are going to say. Make sure that when you are public speaking, you say the material in the way that *you* speak. Anne Temple, who filled in for me because I attended my father-in-law's funeral the day of the Monsanto shareholders' meeting in 2016, told me she walked around her apartment probably fifty times saying, "Mitigate the inevitable!" before the meeting. When she got up to speak, she was comfortable and clear.

Of course, I always recommend omitting any profanity or taking the Lord's name in vain to avoid offending anyone. No matter how passionate you are about your topic, it is just not appropriate to curse during an informational talk.

Practice until you are familiar with the flow of the words. Does the speech flow easily, or does it jump around? Is it sequential in describing the process, topic, or events? Even for a wedding toast—start off when the groom or bride was a baby, work up to elementary school, teenage years, and then college. People relax and can understand the topic better when they can make sense of the flow. It all moves in the same direction—toward what we hope is a happy ending. Or, tell the audience ahead of time which topics you are going to discuss. Then they feel that there will be an order to the talk that may not be chronological but will be in order by topic. When your talk flows, it makes sense—and when it makes sense, people can hear and absorb the information you are giving them. You provide an opportunity to transform the health of their families.

> **Public Speaking Tips**
>
> Exercise the 5 P's:
>
> Prior
> Planning
> Prevents
> Poor
> Performance
>
> Plus: Practice and be Present!

Practice until you are tuned into the timing. If I don't have enough time and get cut short, or if I go over time and take up another speaker's time, I feel unprofessional. The anticipation of feeling unprofessional can make me rush in my talks and speak too quickly. I often find I am rushing because I have not practiced my talk enough and pared it down to what will fit comfortably in the time allotted. This is by far the biggest challenge for me now in public speaking. Once I really get present to what matters to me and I get the information down, delivering accurate scientific information with passion is not the problem for me—it's delivering too much. You can prevent this by practicing and timing yourself.

After you practice and feel that you are comfortable with the words, familiar with the flow, and tuned into the timing, you are ready for the next step—being present.

Be Present

Being an engaging and effective public speaker means being present. Not looking down and reading the paper in front of you but connecting with the audience and looking into their eyes. You are generating energy, delivering important information, making choices to pause or raise your voice, and making eye contact simultaneously. That sounds hard, but it is actually easy when you know your materials and get yourself out of the way. It is one of the most exciting and fulfilling things I have ever done. Every time it feels new, and I feel alive. I love it.

Being present means not worrying about you—how you look, if they like you, or anything else. You can just be completely present to them. Are they getting this information? Is it making a difference for them? Are their eyes lighting up? How can you say this next part to really move them?

Being present also means allowing yourself to feel. If you are moved and choke up, let yourself be. Be present to the emotion that motivated you to speak in the first place. When you share about your family, *feel* your love for them. Your eyes might well up with tears when you really get present to how much you love them. That's okay. If you allow yourself to be present when you talk about a triumph in your cause or thank your supporters, your eyes might well up with tears again. That's even better. Showing real emotion makes you relatable. Be real.

Being a public speaker is giving yourself in service to the public—it is an honor and a privilege. Public speaking is a self-expression of what matters most to you. It is not scary. It's freeing.

CHAPTER TEN
IN THE LION'S DEN

"Never be afraid to raise your voice for honesty and truth and compassion against injustice and lying and greed. If people all over the world . . . would do this, it would change the earth."
—WILLIAM FAULKNER

NOT LONG AFTER the first parades in 2013. I began envisioning speaking directly to the CEO of Monsanto, Hugh Grant (no, not the actor). Although I could not imagine a situation in which that would be possible, I became determined to do so. In the fall of 2014, Alexis Baden-Mayer of Organic Consumers Association called me and said that she thought I should speak at the Monsanto shareholders' meeting. My whole body froze as I listened to her describe how it would work. John Harrington of Harrington Investments owned enough stock—at least $2,500 worth—to be able to present a referendum to change company policy, and I could speak on his behalf. I would get three minutes in front of the entire Monsanto shareholders' meeting. I could speak directly to the CEO, Hugh Grant.

I was terrified and thrilled. Being afraid of looking bad was suddenly larger than life. But when someone asks you to speak, I believe that as long as you are able, you need to say yes—no matter how scared you are. Obviously, they feel you can offer something. So, give it. A week later, I received the generous request from Harrington Investments and it was all arranged. I would be able to say whatever I wanted (of course Harrington Investments would review my talk) as long as I asked the shareholders to vote for the referendum at stake. The referendum was a reasonable one. It was to allow the shareholders to vote for a board member to be placed on the board—for instance, a farmer or pediatrician. Monsanto is the largest "sustainable agriculture company" in the world, claiming to be feeding the world. Wouldn't it make sense for them to have a farmer or pediatrician on their board?

I spent weeks writing and drafting the three-minute talk. Every word was crucial. Every second mattered. I could not go over the three minutes, as I knew I would likely be cut off. I had several people review my talk—a scientist, a farmer, a lawyer, and several moms. I felt a huge responsibility to say everything that any mom who had this opportunity would want to say. I was very aware that this was not about me. It was about what any mom in the world would want Monsanto to know.

Finally, the day had come. The sounds of the boisterous rally that Alexis Baden-Mayor and the Organic Consumers Association (OCA) had organized faded behind me as I walked toward building A of Monsanto headquarters in Saint Louis, Missouri, for the shareholders' meeting. The security officer who was stationed on the perimeter of the property, without a word having passed between us, relayed my pending arrival to the headquarters. "Ms. Honeycutt approaching building A." The staff inside also knew me by name and greeted me cordially. I felt tense and the situation felt surreal, but when a Lego fell out of my hand as I emptied my coat pockets during the security check, I chuckled with the security guard and I was reminded of why I was there—for my sons—for all children—and I felt more focused and at ease. After clearing security and receiving my shareowner sticker, I was escorted to a conference room where Lisa from the nonprofit SumofUs was also sitting. I later learned that SumofUs was a shareholder activist group and speaking at shareholders' meetings was one of the primary objectives of their group. I had no idea that what I was doing was a "thing." To me, it was all new.

I wondered, though, why I was being sequestered in a room with a fellow activist instead of being brought to the conference room. As if reading my mind, the security officer explained that the conference room wasn't ready yet. Still, I thought it was odd that I was not able to be out in the hallway, or near other shareholders.

Several minutes later, a woman walked in, looked right at me, and said, "I am Zen's host." I soon learned that "handler" would have been a better term for her. The staff were prepared. Around 12:50 p.m., we were joined by a few other people, though no one spoke readily. There was another "host" for Lisa, who made sure to steer the conversation cheerily to where people are from.

My host was a mom of fourteen-year-old and ten-year-old boys, a nineteen-year employee, and a self-proclaimed "Monsanto brat." Her father worked at Monsanto for thirty-five years. At 1:00 p.m., we were escorted to the conference room, and along the way she made a concerted effort to engage in conversation. As we passed the cafeteria however, I stopped the chit-chat about our sons' sports and asked her if the cafeteria served organic food. She seemed to expect the question and immediately answered, "Only if no other source is available. For instance, sometimes the only mixed greens or spinach available is organic. Otherwise it is all conventional, and when sweet corn is in season we have GMO sweet corn and it is fabulous." As much as I wanted to, I did not comment.

We entered the enormous shareholders' meeting room. Approximately a thousand people were in the room and when it came time for the meeting to start, every seat was filled. I was brought to the middle of the room where there was a wide aisle. I chose to sit directly in line with Hugh Grant's chair on the stage and behind the microphone. I was assuming my handler would leave me there with Lisa but no, she sat down beside me, and as she did so, my hopes of leaving my phone on and turning on the recording or video disappeared. We had received a notice as we drove in explaining exactly what would be allowed and not allowed in the room and that recording, including with our cell phones, was forbidden. We were reminded as such again before the meeting and again as the meeting started. So as much as I wanted to share this experience with our supporters, I chose not to invite a lawsuit or further trouble later. With great disappointment, I turned my phone off when requested and I could sense my handler relax beside me.

Within a few minutes, Hugh Grant, the CEO of Monsanto—the 2015 Most Hated Corporation in America—approached to greet me. He was a large, bald, stocky man, who could clearly be intimidating. I refused to be intimidated however, or at least to look like I was. I remembered the advice I got from a seasoned leader in our cause: "Smile and look like you are having fun." I smiled and shook his hand. Then I looked him in the eye and said, "You know, Mr. Grant, Moms Across America looks forward to the day when Monsanto no longer makes products that harm our children."

His response (which I cannot write verbatim, risk any mistakes, and open myself up to a lawsuit) challenged my assertion that their products cause harm, implying that they had science on their side. His thick Scottish accent would have been charming had I not known many people who have been harmed from Monsanto's products like Agent Orange, DDT, and Roundup.

I said, "We have science on our side, too, that your products cause harm.

Just consider that if you are wrong, the consequences to the public are enormous." He pointed out that if I was wrong, I was worrying an awful lot of people.

I returned that if I was wrong—which I was not—then the only consequence to the public was that they would be eating organic food. And there was nothing wrong with organic.

As soon as I said that last part about there being nothing wrong with organic, however, I regretted it. An enemy would make sure that there was something wrong with organic to eliminate competition. I prayed they would not go to those lengths. Sadly, however, Monsanto and GMO proponents do not have to try very hard to contaminate organic; drift, rain, irrigation water, and manure from animals that have eaten GMO and glyphosate sprayed grains are being identified as sources of widespread contamination by farmers. It is a common war tactic to eliminate the choices and box in an opponent. It is also another reason why we must not only grow, buy, and eat, organic—but protect it, too.

I wanted him to know I knew he could do better. I looked him in the eye and felt these words flow through me, "You know, Mr. Grant, it takes a big man to create a big and powerful company. It takes an even bigger man to acknowledge when something is not working and change direction."

For one fraction of a second, eye to eye, I saw recognition. I saw a human being who was actually considering what I had to say. I think he got it. His assistant touched his sleeve, he parted with a usual courtesy, and walked away.

The meeting began. I fumed as I watched the fancy videos that used the concept of "Food is Love" that was used in the GMO labeling commercial and was now being used to convince the shareholders how wonderful their products were. I gritted my teeth when the speeches extolled the virtues of the CEO and the Monsanto staff. Then it was my turn. Hugh Grant announced me. My entire body buzzed with energy when I stepped to the microphone in the middle of a thousand people and presented the proxy. Media cameras lined the walls, and everyone was staring at me. I read my statement:

> My name is Zen Honeycutt and I am representing John Harrington of Harrington Investments. We are asking for shareholder support for item number five, shareowner proxy access—an essential mechanism for accountability supported by institutional investors and the SEC.
>
> As the founder of Moms Across America, I was asked to speak

on behalf of millions of mothers.

One out of two children in America today have a chronic illness such as asthma, allergies, autism, autoimmune disease, cancer, obesity, and diabetes. These conditions and more can be directly linked to GMOs and glyphosate—to Monsanto's products.

I am here to say on behalf of struggling parents, **stop poisoning** our children! Glyphosate—a patented antibiotic—has been detected in the air, water, food, our children's urine, our breast milk, Fruit Loops, and in nutrients fed to children with cancer, at levels *far above* what has been shown to destroy *gut bacteria*—where 70 percent of the immune system lies.

Shareholders must know that without proper gut bacteria, our bodies cannot make tryptophan, melatonin, or serotonin. Serotonin regulates insulin—and therefore diabetes, which is on course to bankrupt US health care in thirteen years.

Without serotonin and melatonin, our bodies cannot prevent insomnia, depression, anxiety, and bipolar disorder. Fifty-seven point seven million Americans have mental illness today.

When the gut bacteria are destroyed, food particles and pathogens escape through the intestines, causing allergies and autoimmune diseases. Allergy ER visits have increased 265 percent since GMOs.

Glyphosate is a:

- DNA mutagen and cell disintegrator allowing toxins into the brain.

- A chelator, causing mineral deficiency and the inability to fight cancer.

- An endocrine disruptor, causing infertility, sterility, miscarriages, and birth defects.

I am submitting hundreds of testimonials from mothers describing what Monsanto products are doing to their children and showing that our children get better when they get off GMOs and glyphosate.

I submit studies and papers today showing how glyphosate impacts the gut brain connection, leading to Parkinson's, non-Hodgkin lymphoma, Alzheimer's, Celiac's, autism, and more. Based on our current diagnosis, we can expect that in twenty years, 50 percent of our children will be born with autism.

I understand no one wants to believe this is true, but has anyone on this board seen the newest studies and reports?

What if the very investments shareholders are making to **build** a foundation of security for our children and grandchildren are the same investments that are ***destroying*** their future? What if instead of creating health and prosperity, you are causing ***economic ruin***?

What if instead of trying to help feed millions of people with GMOs, you are in fact hurting ***generations to come***? Mothers say, ***stop it***. ***Stop it now.***

You can make a difference that will alter the future of ***your*** family and ***our*** country. Vote yes on Proxy 5 and vote a pediatrician onto this board. Have the courage to create a new future for Monsanto and America. Thank you.

It was simply a dream come true that I was able to say what I said not just directly to the CEO of Monsanto, but also to the majority of the shareholders and the entire board. It was one of the most fulfilling, thrilling, and terrifying experiences of my life.

When I had finished, the CEO said something to the extent that I had addressed many different issues and that he would respond now to some, but we could address the others later, as I was welcome to get up to ask questions multiple times if I wished. I knew what he was doing. He was trying to appear undaunted by me. The cooler he could play it, the more confidence his shareholders and board would have in him. That's fine, I thought. I can play that game, too. I did not get upset. When I sat down, I heard the room break out in murmurings.

After a series of reports by different executives, they voted on the proxies. I was utterly amazed to hear that our proxy had passed by 53 percent. This was unheard of and unexpected. Shareholder activist proxies only ever got 2–19 percent at most. There were gasps, and scattered applause broke out around the room. I felt actual pats on my back. I could not believe it. I almost cried into my hands. It was truly amazing.

The proxy was advisory, not compulsory, which meant the company was not legally obliged to adopt the suggestions. When Lisa of SumofUs asked if they would honor the wishes of the shareholders, Mr. Grant hemmed and hawed in a typically political fashion. I tried not to let it get me down. We would celebrate our win no matter how small.

I was very nervous about the open Q and A at the end of the shareholder meeting. I had not prepared any statements or questions. I followed my husband's advice to just be present. *Listen for what needs to be addressed. Trust yourself. You don't need to write anything down—you got this*, he said. He was right.

I addressed many different claims, pointed out the flaws, and held them to account in a manner in which I have no regrets. When I felt compelled to get up for the fourth time, people around me chuckled a bit, like, "There she goes again."

I said that I wanted to address the EPA studies. I pointed out that Mr. Grant had mentioned there are studies going back forty years showing the safety of glyphosate. Well, I said, I have seen those studies—and they don't all show safety. For instance, one study on oysters showed that after four days, *the majority of the oysters were closed and not feeding*. Well, what happened on the fifth day? And closed and not feeding . . . isn't that like a coma? How does that prove safety?

At this point, I was no longer addressing Hugh Grant at all. I was looking at the shareholders. I was making eye contact and addressing them personally. I wanted them to get my authenticity. I wanted them to understand that I was not just an angry mother. I was an informed citizen, and they needed to listen and make changes.

I described how another study showed that white shrimp died after four days at levels of glyphosate in the water that were below what is allowed in our food. A recent study showed that glyphosate did not biodegrade, as the company once claimed it did. In fact, it remained viable in dark salt water for 351 days. What is in our wombs? Dark, salty water. How big is a six-week-old fetus? The size of a shrimp. I paused and looked a directly at them.

I saw the gears turning in their heads and I saw faces change with the realization that I might be saying something relevant that shouldn't be ignored. I shared how the pig study in Denmark with thirty thousand pigs clearly showed how, when pigs were fed glyphosate sprayed grains, their miscarriages increased to 30 percent. In contrast, when they did not eat glyphosate, miscarriages went down to 3 percent, then back up to 30 percent with glyphosate sprayed grains . . . at levels *below* what we eat on our food. I said that we currently have the highest rate of infertility and sterility in recorded history—30 percent.

I turned to Hugh Grant and told him that he cannot ignore this. "With the widespread contamination of our water, urine, breast milk, Fruit Loops, and feeding tube liquid, you must be responsible for ways to cut back exposure to our children. Roundup use increased in 2013 by 73 percent. Why? *Because it's not working.* Farmers are using more Roundup to kill the same weeds!" Some farmers get it, though. One, for instance, is an Amish Farmer named John Kempf who said that at his farmers' conference of 150 farmers two years before, when asked who used Roundup, every single farmer raised their hands. This year only eight did. They understand that Roundup is not working for their soil. It destroys the microbes.

"Can you not see the correlation between destroying the microbes in the soil and the good bacteria in the gut?" I asked. "Without healthy soil, we don't have healthy plants or gut bacteria or healthy people. In addition, the use of Roundup has increased because of the encouragement to spray Roundup as a drying agent at harvest!"

It was flowing out of my mouth almost without thought. I have spoken so many times about this topic that it was automatic. I was passionately making my case. I felt UNSTOPPABLE.

I told them that wheat, peas, dry beans/legumes, sugar, and other crops are reportedly being sprayed with glyphosate upon harvest to speed up the harvesting process. So, it's not being sprayed just on GMOs. Unless you are eating organic food, you are likely exposing yourself and your children to levels of glyphosate far above what has been shown to destroy gut bacteria. So, considering the widespread contamination, would you at least advise farmers to stop spraying Roundup as a drying agent?

To my best recollection, Grant said something about how Roundup has the function of being useful in wet areas where fungus or pathogens grow in the crops when they are damp. But then I heard him say that Roundup is recommended to be used as a *weed killer* on crops before harvest.

Interesting. "So, Roundup is *not* recommended as a drying agent to be sprayed before harvest?"

He said something to the extent of—as legal advisors would say—the question has been answered. Roundup is recommended to be used as a *weed killer* on crops before harvest.

I wanted him to say it. "So, Roundup is *not* recommended as a drying agent?"

He replied that this was the third time we had addressed this and that it was time to move on to the next person who had a question. He would not put himself or the company in a position to have it on the record that his company recommends spraying Roundup as a drying agent. It is interesting to note that since then we have seen agricultural advisors warn farmers in online news journals that they cannot say they are using Roundup as a desiccant—that its sole use is for weed killing before harvest.

My favorite moment by far was not when I was speaking, but when a farmer got up and said, "If not Roundup, what then? Will it be something more toxic? Be careful what you ask for."

I was thrilled that someone was asking, "If not Roundup, what then?" *Yes!* They were wondering! That was all we need for the farmers to do—to get to that place where they were looking for alternatives.

I hoped that farmers would begin to see that they had been misled. Farmers are not to be vilified. They are working tirelessly. They are devoted to doing a thankless job for the good of the people. It is the EPA and chemical companies that must be held accountable for misleading farmers, landscapers, and citizens around the world.

In the following year, 2016, I arranged for three women—Beth Savitt of the Shaka Movement from Maui, Rachel Parent of Kid's Right to Know, Canada, and Anne Temple (who spoke in my place) of Moms Across America—to return to the meeting, and all three women spoke passionately in front of one thousand shareholders and asked questions. They were limited this time, however, to one question. The following year I returned with Anne. This time, the meeting had about sixty people in it and the recording was not made available to shareholders. I told them, "I would have been here last year but on the day of the meeting I was at the funeral of my father-in-law, who used Roundup and died of liver disease. I am back this year with a study proving that Roundup causes liver disease." I saw the look of dread in the board members' eyes in the first row, but I looked directly at them and I continued with my three-minute talk.

This kind of confrontation is something Monsanto wants to avoid. They now take votes before the speaker's presentation for a referendum, not afterwards, making the speaker's presentation ineffectual. Since this meeting in 2015, a federal bill has been proposed that would make it legal under federal law to limit the ability for shareholders to present proxies altogether and have the shareholder meeting held remotely, via a webinar, instead of in person. This would allow the host corporations to control who gets to speak, and for how long, in a much more restricted manner. At the time of the writing of this book, anyone who owns just one share can go to the shareholders' meeting of a company and ask a two- to three-minute question in front of all the shareholders—except for Virginia and Delaware, which made changes in 2017 and allow remote annual meetings. The new federal bill would limit proposals and rob shareholders and the citizens who speak on their behalf—like me—of the opportunity to gain time and attention before the shareholders.

This is another example of corporate control taking far too much power within our government.

Dow, DuPont, and Syngenta Shareholders' Meetings

When I visited other chemical company giants, I had very different experiences.

There was no protest and no supporters at the Dow shareholder meeting in Michigan. I was all alone. I had help getting there, though, from Samuel, a thirty-year former bioengineering employee of Dow with the utmost pride in his company, who allowed me to attend the meeting on his behalf. Their mission to feed the world is on the right track, he said to me, and he does not agree with my opinion. He does support the right of free speech, however, so he helped me. That generous act speaks volumes of the kind of man he is and the kind of country we could be if we all supported such free speech and had an open mind to hear each other's opinions. I was touched. I made sure to tell him I would share his values with my sons. At dinner later, I shared with my sons what Samuel did, and their mouths made little O's of surprise. They learned that despite our perspectives, we can all still honor each other. Samuel reminded me that we can all be great, and I will be grateful to him forever. His former CEO, however, was not so generous.

The Dow CEO was not allowing questions on any other topics other than what was on the agenda, so I had to think on a dime and make my comments fit their topics. It was stressful, and I was upset that I did not get more time.

Afterward, a shareholder assured me that I had gotten my point across and that they were shamed enough to know that they needed to change direction, away from the toxins. A sustainability director at Dow approached me, asking to speak with me at the end of the meeting. We talked about the technology that they had been developing that cleaned up oil and pollutants in seawater, and I felt a spark of hope. A former Dow employee approached me in the parking lot, telling me story after story about sickness in her family, how cancer was rampant in her city, and how appreciative she was that I spoke up. With earnest pleading she said, "Please do not give up." I held her hands as tears welled up in her eyes.

"I will never give up," I said. I knew it had been worth the trip.

The day after the Dow meeting in Michigan, I attended the DuPont shareholders' meeting in Maryland and there was much pomp and circumstance—bright lights, a giant timer, splashy videos, and the CEO behaved like Tony Robbins. It was a show. I wasn't the only activist in the room at DuPont. At least a dozen others got up and asked questions about toxic waste sites that DuPont was not taking responsibility for, pollution, cancer clusters, accusations of the theft of intellectual property . . . it was clear that these people had been coming every year for many years—some for decades. All these people had suffered from the actions of this big chemical company, and none of them were getting satisfaction. I realized why DuPont had to try so hard to look good. The reality was—and is—very, very bad.

Unfortunately, I found out the day before the Syngenta shareholders' meeting in Switzerland that I might not be allowed entry into the meeting. I told my mom supporters and they began calling and emailing the headquarters, asking them to let me in. I was up until 2:00 a.m., woke up at 6:00 a.m. and jet lag had me feeling like I was walking with lead feet. At the headquarters, after not being allowed by the clerk to register, I was directed to speak with the head of the legal department. After much back and forth, I was only allowed to meet with three heads of research and development and communications in a separate building.

The heads of the departments were all women. I surprised them when I pointed out the perfect profit circle created by chemical companies making people sick and then their sister companies making people "better." They scoffed and denied that Syngenta was involved in such a scenario. I refuted that statement by pointing out that Syngenta's sister company, AstraZeneca, made over four hundred drugs that directly treated symptoms shown to have been caused by pesticides. They were silenced. They looked visibly shaken. It was hard for me to believe, however, that they did not already know this.

I made the same request of the Syngenta staff as I did of the CEOs of

Monsanto, Dow, and DuPont—namely, to change direction away from the toxins. These three women appeared to listen much more intently. I could see their gears turning, and they responded in a thoughtful manner. I was grateful to have discourse with them. I was surprised to learn at the end of the year that Syngenta stated that they intentionally sold less glyphosate. In some cases, less is more. In this case, none is better.

It was reported by Carey Gillam, for the *St. Louis Dispatch* on May 5, 2015:

> The EPA's upcoming draft risk assessment on glyphosate comes at a time when Monsanto and other agrichemical companies are developing biopesticides, which are based on natural organisms like plant and soil microbes rather than synthetic chemicals and seen by some as alternatives to traditional pesticides. Jim Jones, assistant administrator for the EPA Office of Chemical Safety and Pollution Prevention, said the EPA is encouraging development of biopesticides because they "have very favorable human health and environmental profiles." He said they are likely to overtake synthetic chemicals in agriculture at some point if their use continues what he called "dramatic" growth.

Reading this article, I rejoiced about the move away from synthetic chemicals, while feeling healthy skepticism about the biopesticides.

Getting over the fear of public speaking and standing up for what is right is an action that makes not only you UNSTOPPABLE but also adds to the momentum of your entire cause. Others are encouraged and feel that their time and effort mean something when one of their own stands up and says what they want said. That is why we cheer speakers at a rally! The outcome of your mission—generations of good health—means far more than looking good for a few minutes. Risk looking bad. Stand up, speak up, and share your heart.

Corporate Agenda

Keep in mind when you get tired and want to stop that Monsanto, Syngenta, Bayer, BASF, Dow, and DuPont are not stopping. They are trying to merge into larger corporations and get stronger. You children are still growing. Your neighbor still has weeds he wants to spray with weed killer. Your family still needs to eat, and choices about food need to be made every day. Rest first, snuggle with your kids, and kiss your spouse. Then get up and keep going. Keep learning. Most importantly, reach out to someone else who is doing something to make our food supply and towns safer, and just listen to them and support them. You will be so inspired when you are around someone else who is taking action. I promise that you will find the strength to keep going.

In spring of 2016, Monsanto proudly announced that they had invested $975 million in a new production facility in Louisiana for the production of Dicamba—their replacement for glyphosate—and they had plans to build a facility in Arizona. Even though four states placed bans on Dicamba-based herbicides in the spring of 2017, the EPA continues to allow its use, and Monsanto continues to ask farmers to run on their toxic treadmill of chemical cocktails to feed their shareholder profits. In the summer of 2017, Monsanto announced an expanded partnership with Valent U.S.A. LLC in the 2018 Roundup Ready PLUS Crop Management Solutions platform. They have a whole batch of "new and improved" herbicides to sell farmers. They continue to think that more and more toxic chemicals will suppress weeds.

However, it's not just the thirty-eight weeds currently resistant to glyphosate herbicides that are a problem for farmers. During the past forty years of chemical farming, with the past twenty being the most intense, the microbes in the soil have been severely depleted as a result of the chemicals. In some areas, such as the United Kingdom, they project that their topsoil will no longer be viable within thirty to forty years, less than two generations. So now, Monsanto is genetically engineering and patenting microbes in the soil. They plan to make money from the mess they created.

The chemical companies' agenda is to sell as many chemical products and patented GMO seeds as they can, thereby controlling both the food supply and the market on chemicals. To do this, they must silence the opposition. I witnessed this firsthand in 2015 when I went to Iowa to attend the Norman E. Borlaug International Symposium, known informally as the *Borlaug Dialogue*—where they hand out the World Food Prize to the favorite

GMO supporter of the year. I felt like a tiger swimming in a pool of sharks. The conference is a giant GMO love fest, with plenty of government agency department heads like the USDA and FDA, and CEOs of corporations like Google, Starbucks, Monsanto, Dow, DuPont, banks like the Bank of Africa, dignitaries like the President of Malawi, and nonprofits like the Bill and Melinda Gates Foundation. In the first, smaller panel I attended, I brought up the UN's report, referred to as "Wake Up Before It's Too Late: Organic Food is the Only Way to Feed the World," and the report was dismissed as a bunch of "opinions." The tension in the room was palpable. I was physically blocked by a woman in a suit from approaching the panelists afterward, until I looked the woman in the eye and questioned her . . . she then stepped aside. Later, in the main room, when Chelsea Clinton, a representative from the Bill and Melinda Gates Foundation, and the CTOs and CEOs of Monsanto, Starbucks, and Google took the stage before one thousand people, they got clever. They announced they would not be taking questions by microphone. They were "going modern" and would be taking questions by Twitter only. They were preventing me from going to the microphone. They were afraid of what I might say. So I proceeded to Tweet question after question about Roundup and birth defects and cancer. I could see from the disgust on the face of the moderator that the panelists were clearly disturbed by my questions . . . and they completely ignored them.

At the *Borlaug Dialogue,* I also saw the chemical companies' agenda to brainwash our students about the "benefits" of GMOs in action. Otherwise brilliant high school and college students, flown in on scholarships, parroted the chemical companies' talking points with pride. One college student—I will call her Sadie—who sat next to me confided in me that her teacher at a major Midwestern university actually admitted to getting bonuses for every student who signed up to major in agriculture. Even though Sadie clearly expressed that she wanted to be a veterinarian, she had been pressured by her professor to attend the *Borlaug Dialogue* and embrace GMOs. Elementary school youth are being brainwashed as well. Numerous photos on Facebook have popped up, showing the GMO propaganda that is being slipped into our youth's science programs, due to the federal education laws that allow corporate funding for our public schools. If we are not aware of their agenda and do not take action, the next generation will be brainwashed.

Many people have asked why the chemical companies are allowed to continue doing what they are doing. How can they sleep at night? The answer to both questions is money. And the only way they will stop is if they do not continue to make money. They will simply keep going until what they are doing is no longer economically viable. One should understand that some employees at Monsanto do not see what they do as greedy or evil. They believe the management, who present themselves as noble and present Monsanto as a company bringing technology to the world that is critical for survival. The management, however, is legally obligated to provide profits for their shareholders. Once they invest in a technology, it almost doesn't matter if that technology doesn't work the way they thought it would. They need to find a way to make it work somehow, or some other country that will allow it, in order to recoup their investment and be profitable. This is why even though DDT has been banned in the United States, it is still sold in third world countries. This is why Monsanto is targeting Africa as the new frontier for GMO seeds . . . lots of land, lots of people, and no previous experience with all the negative impacts of GMOs. I shudder to think what will happen to their land, water, and children should they allow toxic GMO chemical farming to infiltrate all of Africa.

Alice Gleeson from Uganda, whom I met in Australia while on speaking tour for two weeks in Australia and New Zealand, allowed me to interview her about the impact of the trial GMO crops in her home village. In the video, found under "Resources" at www.momsacrosstheworld.org, Alice blows every argument Monsanto has about the benefits of GMOs out of the water in fourteen minutes without even being aware of doing so. She just tells her story about her mother, father, sister, and village experiencing diabetes, sickness, and death—due, she believes, to the chemicals from her family's farm. Alice herself had nine miscarriages until she eliminated processed GMO food and milk from her diet. She then gave birth to three healthy children in her late thirties. Because Monsanto's chemicals destroyed the soil, after a few years the villagers were unable to grow the variety of crops they used to grow and began to starve. GMO corn in her village was not the boon they were promised. In fact, it was a death sentence.

Alice told me her story because she wanted the harm and death to stop. She loved her people—all people—and she wanted us to be safe and healthy.

Alice shared with me that she had previously attended Dr. Vandana Shiva's presentation and afterward she asked her who would stand up to Monsanto in Uganda. Vandana had said, "You. Now. You need to be the leader." She didn't say, "If you feel like it," or, "When you have time." The time is now.

CHAPTER ELEVEN

AGAINST ALL ODDS
Transforming Conflict

"Darkness cannot drive out darkness; only light can do that. Hate cannot drive out hate; only love can do that."
—MARTIN LUTHER KING, JR.

WHEN YOU START connecting with communities and working toward a common goal, it's not all holding hands and singing "Kumbaya." There are many very eccentric people that are also very passionate and committed to activists' causes that you will be working with. You can't take their commitment but leave out the eccentricities. You also just don't know, in today's world of anonymous internet interactions, who is who and what is real. Anyone can say anything. People are much more likely to criticize each other when they are hiding behind a screen. So, when you put yourself out there, expect eccentric people, passionate people, *even people on your side,* to take exception to what you have to say or the actions you take . . . and be set upon transforming conflict and fears no matter what.

Fear grew in my heart when it appeared that a group of masked hacktivists was going to join in the Fourth of July parades with us Moms. They saw it as an opportunity to protest Monsanto and were planning on wearing sinister looking black and white masks in the parades. My alarm bells went off. I checked with our supporters.

Our MAA mothers were not happy about this. "What if they wear their shirts that say F**k Monsanto in front of my six-year-old?" "I am not comfortable with masked people around my kids." "This is not a protest. We will not be allowed back next year if a bunch of masked people show up with us,

Zen," they said. "Our website does not show any masked people." "We don't promote skull and crossbones."

We were all in alignment, except in terms of how to handle the situation. One of my mom supporters begged me to speak to one of the leaders of a group that might join in and have her ask the hacktivists not to wear masks or skull and crossbones shirts, or to drop F-bombs. The request was to keep it family friendly. I did not want to do this. I did not want to ask *someone else* to make a request for me about the event I had instigated. It felt weak and wimpy. Against my better judgment, I did what this mom asked of me. It was my choice—but in hindsight, I see now that it was not the best choice.

I called the leader and she did not like what I was asking. She felt it was excluding people. She felt it was not in the spirit of America the Free. She did not want to do it. By this point, my spidey sense was tingling like mad. I sighed and, with deep hesitation, asked her to do it anyway. I asked her to let them know that this event was different. It was not a protest—it was an all-American celebration—and protesting simply wasn't appropriate. I made the analogy that when going to someone's backyard barbeque, you don't show up protesting. We had different perspectives. She disagreed with the principle of what I was asking. She saw it as censorship, and when she posted her request it was not good. She made the request, but you could tell she was not happy about it (at least she was authentic), and it created a sh*t storm.

All of a sudden, I was getting threats of violence from around the world. *"F**k you!"* "If I ever see you I will throw a brick at your head," "We could erase your life, be warned," and more. The messages had crossed the line from opposition to the cause to opposition to *me*. The words affected me in a real, physical way. I experienced severe fatigue. I feared for my family's safety and my life. They tried to find links between my husband's employer—a health-care medical device company—and Monsanto. My husband, an IT guy who managed software and had no connection to Monsanto, feared for his job and thus his ability to keep our family sheltered and fed.

The hacktivists began investigating us and they dug up that at one point in time, Monsanto bought medical devices and lab tests from my husband's employer. They posted a Facebook page called World War Z(en), which was a take on a zombie apocalypse movie, with pictures of my husband's and my faces over the actors' faces, fleeing the scene of burning, collapsing buildings with his company logo photoshopped on them. They posted pictures of me as a dominatrix and called me a narcissistic cult leader.

To our shock and dismay, we learned that, unfortunately, one of the devices sold by his company was the gene gun used to make many GMOs. It was also used to research Alzheimer's and leukemia. But still, it was as if they had the "smoking gun." I thought, "This is it. People are going to be so upset that they are not going to want to be affiliated with Moms Across America, and this will affect the cause as a whole." I was devastated. My heart filled with dread and anger.

I got angry with my husband when he said he didn't know that his company sold lab equipment to Monsanto. I wasn't sure I believed him. Then I got angry because these hacktivists were affecting my marriage.

Some might not think about the reality that thousands of companies (in addition to Monsanto) bought medical devices from his company. By the same token, thousands of other companies (not just his) sold products to Monsanto, and it didn't mean they were in collusion with them. Did the hacktivists assume that the office supply stores, coffee, and copier companies that sold Monsanto their products were "in bed" with Monsanto?

I still felt that Moms Across America could somehow lose credibility over my husband's supposed link to Monsanto. I had to constantly manage the Facebook page, where threat after threat was being posted and accusations poured in under posts that were hidden in the comments.

I began to get sick. I lost seventeen pounds over the next month or so, and ended up weighing only 113 pounds. I had anxiety every night, couldn't sleep, and often had heart palpitations. We feared my husband might lose his job when the hacktivists threatened to take down his company. He had to tell his bosses. They put their security team on it and found many more attacks than the ones of which we were aware. These people were serious. They were pissed off. They felt they were being censored. I completely understood but censoring them was not my intention. We just wanted to have our event be the way we Moms envisioned. I struggled with fear, regret, and anxiety. My stomach was constantly twisted and tight.

As my family and I were driving across the country for the first parade events, to the Fourth of July parade in Connecticut, passing GMO fields of corn and handing out flyers to moms' groups, I had to continually find an internet hot spot, check my Facebook page, and delete comments. As a result of being stressed about these attacks, I did not video blog or post regularly about the trip. It was a loss for me and our supporters, who could have been encouraged by our interactions across the country with organic farmers and supporters. I did not tell anyone about the ordeal with the hacktivists because I did not want to bring attention to the drama. I wanted everyone to stay focused on creating successful groups in parades. I told only the mom who urged me to make that call that put this all into motion. She was upset. I completely understood why the leader did what she did. What we were asking went against what she stood for. It was not authentic to her. It was my mistake for asking her to do it in the first place. To this day, I have zero hard feelings toward her. I appreciate her dedication to the cause. At the time, however, I won't lie—it hurt. I am sure there was a great deal of stress for the leader and my mom supporter, too. I was very sorry how it all happened.

It took a long time to resolve things with the hacktivists. After a supporter got wind of threats on a hacktivist Facebook news feed two days before the parades, I had to get my website designer to back up my website and ban spammers to prevent them from "taking out Moms Across America." On the day of the parade, nothing happened. No masked men showed up, and I finally breathed a sigh of relief. A few days after the parades, however, another hacktivist started up again with the supposed Monsanto "connection" and began posting about other partners and supporters. They call it doxing. Several hacktivists research and post everything they can find about a person and draw connections to anything sordid or lacking in integrity. It was like a sci-fi movie. It seemed so surreal when they posted pictures of my home birth—so invasive, and yet irrelevant.

By this time, I honestly could not tell if the doxxers were people paid by Monsanto to argue with me, people who were influenced by people from Monsanto who used to be on my side but suddenly doubted me, or people who were simply on my side and just pissed about not being able to be in the parades. They could have been people who were pretending to be members of the hacktivist group—they could have been anyone.

One of my state leaders, Jessica, saw the posts and said, "Oh no, this stops." She befriended one of the more reasonable sounding hacktivists and discovered she was a homebound woman with health issues. She asked her to ask the other hacktivists to get on Facebook and start a conversation in the form of a thread of private messaging. Then she called me and asked me to get online and "talk" with them. Luckily, my battery was charged, and I had a hot spot.

It was ten o'clock at night and I was alone except for my sleeping children in a partially collapsed tent in Connecticut in the pouring rain. My husband had flown back to California for his job. Water was leaking in a corner a few feet from me and I sat cross-legged on a hump of higher ground with the blue light of the laptop glaring at me. I had Jessica on the phone and the message thread in front of me. They threw accusation after accusation at me. "You don't ever tell us what to do." "Your husband is in bed with Monsanto." "You make money off Monsanto and are controlled by the opposition."

They said I was an infiltrator—meaning I secretly worked *for* Monsanto and was doing their dirty work by getting people to label GMOs instead of banning them. It was incredible. Here I was, working eight to ten hours some days, building a website, calling sponsors for money to pay for flyers, writing flyers and organizing T-shirts, stickers, and materials for a nationwide event . . . volunteering . . . and they thought I was working for the company that was poisoning us all. Incredible. I physically ached to think that anyone could think I was that evil. I ached to think that anyone was that resigned about the world, that darkness of that kind existed at all, and that anyone could be convinced to *be* that kind of resigned and angry. I ached because with every accusation, I felt like I myself was becoming more jaded and losing my light and love—and it terrified me.

It took everything I had to be calm and clear, and stay focused. "I made a request," I said, "that did not come out well. I should never have asked anyone else to make that request for me."

One of the hacktivists started to turn on the leader that I had asked to make the request. Suddenly I was fearful that they would attack her, and I didn't wish that on anyone.

"No, no," I said. "That was my mistake. It was my responsibility. Please do not go after her." They tried to argue with me about that—they really did not want anyone telling them what to do.

"I am sorry you feel like I was telling you what to do and I totally understand why you feel that way. That was not my intention. I wanted you to join us—just not with the masks, swear words, or skull and crossbones shirts. We just wanted this event to feel safe to the moms."

They pointed out that my son wore a skull and crossbones T-shirt in a photo on our cross-country trip. I replied that a ten-year-old wearing a "Game Over" video game symbol was different than a grown man wearing a mask and skull and crossbones shirt at a family parade.

I tried to explain that, like a birthday party with a theme, when you go to someone else's party you dress appropriately. You aren't required to but, like at a prom, people usually wear a tux or a dress. I think they started to see what I was saying.

When they brought up the gene gun I wrote, "That device is also used for Alzheimer's and leukemia research. I have had people in my extended family die of both of those diseases. Have you?" In addition, I pointed out, "A medical device can be used for good or evil, just like a pen . . . or *a Facebook page*." I said, referring to his World War Z(en) page.

Then I felt I needed to acknowledge him. "Very clever, by the way," I wrote.

"LOL," he wrote back.

And suddenly, the tension dropped. We began to talk more about the cause, and less about my husband or me. Soon, after several more statements of how we moms just love our kids, how we want a healthy future, and how we want this particular event to be family friendly, they agreed to remove the Facebook page attacking me and to "stand down."

I sobbed in the night. I yearned for my husband. I felt the anxiety of months of stress begin to drain.

A day or two later, I got a Facebook message with an attachment from the hacktivist group. It contained information about Monsanto that could help our cause. I was shocked. Wow. What a gesture. They wanted to help. All the remaining anxiety left my body and I felt like we were finally on the same side again. I cannot express how glad I was that chapter had ended and for them to tell me that if I ever needed anything, to just ask. What a miracle. The relief that washed over my body soothed months of intense anxiety. I was so grateful I could have kissed the ground that Jessica walked on. I was also extremely glad that I had learned communication skills—specifically to acknowledge people and especially in times of stress or conflict.

> Most people are looking to be acknowledged, loved, or admired. If you can find a way to do this, you can build a bridge of communication and dissolve conflict.

I did not know the legal issues involved with using the information I was given by the hacktivists, however, or how it was obtained, and I did not want to be sued. It was not information about Monsanto's products, but was information about their staff that might no longer be true, so I could not use it with certainty. I suppose others would do differently—especially Monsanto. During Prop 37, suddenly fake "Green Democrat" groups were sending out flyers with *No on 37* checked off and *yes* on everything else a Democrat would likely vote yes on. This was unbeknownst to me at the time—when I was searching my conscience for whether I should use the information I'd been given. Monsanto, meanwhile, was not struggling with any such ethics. According to released discovery documents, they were busy ghostwriting reports and paying scientists to have papers submitted that covered up the harm of glyphosate herbicides for decades. They were also caught paying hundreds of people to work online and counter all opposition . . . like, for instance, me. Many of the people that hurled accusations at me and got the World War Z(en) hacktivist riled up could have been Monsanto employees. I will never know for sure.

I want to be clear—this type of harassment is not going to happen to people who simply sign a petition, share infographics, or even march in a protest. This type of harassment would only happen if you take on serious leadership and make life very difficult for the opposition. In general, nothing will happen to anyone who takes on activism. But after my experience, I believe that even if you are confronted, it is worth it, your role as a leader will keep you going, and you will transform pretty much anything.

Tips for Transforming Conflict

1. Do not expect that people who are "on your side" of a cause will always agree with you. Expect differences. Acknowledge them for what they contribute.

2. If you are going to engage, be curious. Don't assume.

3. In some situations that go beyond just random insults on social media, it could behoove you to be willing to face your critics and have a conversation with the intention of getting to know them and making them feel "gotten." Gotten does not mean that you agree with them—it simply means you get where they are coming from.

4. In times of conflict, remember that listening is key. Seek to understand rather than be understood. Listen for what they need to have said to make a difference for them. You can transform intense struggle into

> freedom and peace together by connecting with "opposition" and becoming friends.
>
> 5. Acknowledge them. Find a way to connect, and you never know what will happen.
>
> 6. One of my favorite mottos is, "We are only one conversation away from creating what we want." What is that conversation?
>
> 7. Above all, do not let anyone from either your side or their side stop you from being an activist. The opposition may have engineered situations and planted people to achieve exactly that.

Hitting Home

In some cases—like hundreds of troll comments on Christmas Eve, website spammers, and an intern who came into my home and, within a few days, threatened a lawsuit against me—it was pretty obvious that the opposition was behind it all. However, sometimes things happen, and it is not clear if the opposition is behind the scenes.

In January 2016, Moms Across America put a billboard up right outside Monsanto's headquarters during the time of their shareholders' meeting that said, "Our children get better when they avoid GMOs and toxins. Invest in the future. Go organic." This one billboard sparked a dream come true—support for a series of nationwide billboard campaigns. The following year, five different billboards went up all across the country that received half a million views per month in each of the 191 locations nationwide.

Two weeks after the first billboard went up, an outside consultant came into my husband's company for a "reorg" of three hundred people. Of the hundreds of employees in his division, my husband was singled out. After fourteen years of good reviews, he was fired with no notice. He came home in shock. We could not prove that Monsanto was behind it, but I knew that Monsanto knew that the only way I was able to volunteer full-time and create Moms Across America without a salary for three years was because of my husband's income. We were determined, however, to see the situation as an opportunity.

Todd had a realization that my mission with Moms Across America was also his mission. Being let go from his position was the best thing that had happened to us in a long time. We made it work in our favor. He dug in, heart and soul. He added search engine optimization (SEO) to his technical skill set. He also started supporting other websites and helping Moms Across America fend off trolls and spammers. Often, on Sunday afternoons, Todd can be found deleting, banning, and blocking spammers from posting porn and live streaming football games to our website. The reason the spammers do this is because it lowers the safety of a website if you have spammers posting such material. Google sends you a warning that they may take you off their search engine. If you do not appear on Google, basically you are in the desert of cyberspace. It is a serious issue to have a secure website and, without my husband's skills and dedication, Moms Across America would probably not have the reach—over 1.5 million a month on just Facebook and Twitter alone—that we have today.

Another suspicious instance was when, a few months after Todd lost his job, on the second day of our National Toxin Free Tour 2016, my entire family and dog were sprayed by helicopter with weed killer. We were volunteering on an organic farm in Utah in a makeshift greenhouse with an open roof. I saw a helicopter spraying chemicals in a field near us. At first, I thought the helicopter was spraying the huge mono crop (likely GMO) farm in the valley below, but then I realized it was spraying the grassy field in between the farm we were volunteering on and the mono crop farm. At the time, I did not know why they were spraying there—the guys with the truck of chemicals that filled the helicopter up time after time were too far away to ask. I filmed the spraying for seven minutes for a live Facebook feed. I was aghast at what I was seeing but I thought that the spraying was far enough away—about a half a mile or more—and I did not want to believe that it would affect us.

I was standing on the top of a hill in a red shirt and big white hat while I was filming. About two hundred feet behind us was our twenty-eight-foot red-and-white striped motorhome with Moms Across America emblazoned across the side. I am sure the pilot of the helicopter saw me. Soon the helicopter looked like it was going to begin to spray closer to my family's position, so I turned off the video and ran into the greenhouse to tell my family that we had to leave. Before I could speak, I heard the huge clamoring of helicopter propellers and saw the sprayers of the helicopter above emitting a white stream of chemicals directly over our heads.

My head screamed in terror, my mouth said, "Get out now! Everyone, we are leaving!" I grabbed my dog and made sure my kids were running beside me. As we left the greenhouse, within seconds, my son Bodee's nose began dripping bright red blobs of blood. I was reeling in shock. I took a picture immediately, feeling that we had to document this—someone had to be held accountable for this.

The helicopter pilot did not stop when he saw us running. In fact, he made another pass. I filmed it, outraged, saying for the recording that I needed to find out immediately what chemical he was spraying. It was odd that I did not say on the video that my family was just directly sprayed. I think I was dazed and confused. But we were sprayed. We were coughing, our throats hurt, our clothes smelled, and my son's nose wouldn't stop bleeding. I sent my family to the RV to prevent them from inhaling any more of the drift. I didn't think to tell them to take their clothes off and shower. I was aware enough, however, to call the owner of the farm. We agreed that we needed to file a police report. The police arrived several minutes later with the man who commissioned the spraying of the chemicals—the head of the Utah Wildlife Resources Division. He looked nervous and stern.

The first thing I asked him was what he had sprayed. He backed up and waved to the truckload of Plateau, a toxic herbicide that contains the active chemical ingredient imazapic. With further investigation after this incident, I learned that a Colorado lawyer who was working to get imazapic banned had stated that it was the most toxic herbicide on the market, causing nerve damage and neurotoxicity.

When I asked the man why he sprayed, he explained that they were trying to eliminate invasive annual weeds so that the perennial weeds could grow and feed the field mice and native fauna.

He said somberly, "We have never sprayed this field before—we probably won't ever spray it again."

"Then *why* today? Why the *one* day that *my family* is here?" I was so angry that I was almost spitting.

His face got red and tight. He sputtered, "I don't know. Bad luck, I guess?" I swear I saw a wave of guilt and shame. I was highly suspicious. My spidey senses were firing like cannons.

I couldn't prove it, but I felt it in my bones that this incident had been intentional.

It wouldn't be the first time that an activist has been targeted in this way, either. I have heard of other activists who have reported low flying planes spraying their properties. I fumed. I couldn't think straight at first. Then the fury of a mother protecting her family came out. I demanded that he see the damage that he had caused and the potential of a lifetime of harmful effects. I asked him if he was willing to pay for my sons' medical bills if they got nerve damage. What would he do about it if they were sterile someday because of these chemicals?

Then the helicopter pilot and tank attendant truck driver swaggered onto the scene. They each looked about twenty-two years old, red eyed, probably high. The pilot was smirking.

"Why are you smiling?" I demanded to know.

"I'm not," he said. "Just doing my job."

I could barely control my rage. Through a clenched jaw I commanded that he acknowledge that this wasn't funny, and that my kids could be impacted for the rest of their lives. He refused. One of the most infuriating moments of the conversation was when he bossed me to stop talking and just fill out the report. He also volunteered the information that if I was going to sue, I would sue *him* not the state of Utah Wildlife Resources Division.

"People have tried four or five times before," he bragged, "but they never win."

Just as expected all of them—the police, the sprayer, truck driver, and the Utah Wildlife Resources Division (WRD) head—all claimed that I should not be upset because the EPA has deemed the chemicals to be safe.

I launched into a lecture that left them stunned. "I just came back last week from meeting with the EPA in Washington, DC," I said, "with a team of scientists. They admitted to me directly that they do not have *one single long-term animal study* on the final formulation with blood analysis showing safety on the world's most widely used herbicides. Not *one*. Why? Because *it is not their policy*. They only require safety studies on the *one* declared active chemical ingredient of the formulation, not the final formulation. So, they don't have safety studies on any pesticides or herbicides—including Plateau. None. So not you," I said pointing at each man, "or you, or you, or you can claim that what you just sprayed on my family is safe with any scientific standing. None."

I was furious. The police officer, WRD head, sprayer, and truck driver all went out to "inspect" the organic field. They looked awfully chummy to me, so I followed. I would not let them have time alone together in their good ol' boys club to dismiss the harm done. The police officer did nothing in the end. He did not arrest the sprayer. The sprayer remained cocky and arrogant. His partner even said, "What do you want us to do, go back to fracking?" It saddened me that some young men in our country feel that the only jobs they can find are ones that poison the earth. At the root of this entire mess of a food system and weed management is the lack of jobs. It's a complicated mess.

Eventually, talking about being sprayed with the perpetrators of the spraying lost its usefulness for me. I became exasperated. We packed up our RV and left to go to the hospital to get checked out. I had no idea if my family was seriously injured, and we needed to find out. Plus, I knew if we were going to sue, going to the hospital would be necessary.

After a battery of simple tests, the doctors deemed us to be "fine" and said there was nothing we could do except take a shower. The situation just got worse and worse. The hospital shower had no hot water—it was icy cold, and we were supposed to shower for twenty minutes. The doctor couldn't test our urine or blood for the chemicals, so I asked if we could collect samples anyway. I knew someone who might be able to test. The hospital staff agreed. We collected our whole family's urine samples in the heavy-duty plastic sample cups provided by the hospital—the ones with the hard, blue tops. You could stand on them and they would not break. (If you sense foreshadowing here, you would be correct.)

We stored those urine cups in our freezer for three weeks while we drove cross-country. They took up valuable space, but I felt it was necessary. Finally, the lab I had contacted to do the testing got back to me. The owner emailed me, saying, "Yes, we can test for imazapic (the declared active chemical ingredient in the weed killer Plateau). Send me your urine samples." So I did.

I expected the lab to receive the samples in two days. Four days later, I got a call from an assistant at the lab. It was a new person I had never spoken with before. She sounded irritated and said something along the lines of, "It looks like you sent us urine samples?"

"Yes," I said, dumbfounded. "I did."

"Why would you send us urine? The box is crushed! It is leaking everywhere!"

"*What?*" I was shocked on both accounts—one, that she did not know *why* we were sending her urine samples and two, because my samples were *crushed.* "*What do you mean* you don't know why I sent you urine samples? I got an email from the owner saying, 'Yes we can test for imazapic. Send me your urine samples.'"

She got quiet, then asked, "What email did you use?"

I told her.

"Oh no . . . that one has been compromised," she said.

I felt like I had been punched in the gut.

"So, the samples were crushed? Can't you save any of the urine to test? Those samples are my only evidence for a lawsuit against a helicopter company for spraying my entire family with weed killer!"

"No," she said. "You can barely tell it was a box. It looks like it was run over—it was completely flattened. It's in a plastic bag and it's leaking everywhere. I am not touching this."

I pleaded with her, but she was angry. She would not let me talk to the owner.

I called the post office and they confirmed that it was crushed before it left the midway station, before arriving at the lab. The postal worker remembered it, but no photos were taken.

I was devastated. I desperately wanted to sue and get some justice for my family. I wanted to prevent this from ever happening again to anyone else. Our only chance of getting some form of media attention (and therefore possibly policy change) by proving that the chemical was in my family had been thwarted. My brain felt scrambled with anger.

A lawyer later told me that even if I had the urine samples, however, that it would have been almost impossible to win against the state of Utah. Apparently, they have a clause in their constitution declaring that the state can basically take actions for the greater good even if doing so violates the rights of individuals. This didn't give me closure. The injustice still hurt. With a willing lawyer licensed to practice in Utah, I would still have pursued a lawsuit.

A few days later, Bernie Sanders was robbed of his nomination, the DNC chaos broke out, and the DARK (Denying Americans the Right to Know) Act was passed partly because the Organic Trade Association threw our cause under the bus by endorsing it, effectively hiding GMOs in our food. I was convinced America was on a freefall from democracy to oligarchy and I slipped into despair.

Not so coincidentally, at this time I threw my back out and was incapacitated for over a week. I couldn't move or even go to the bathroom without help and felt badly about the inconvenience to my husband, but he looked me in the eyes and told me as he helped me, "Zen if I had to do this for the rest of our lives, I would do it." Hearing him say those words filled me with the feeling that I was supported and loved. I needed that. Losing so many battles all at once can make a person feel broken. Family support can make you feel whole again. Be sure to remind your loved ones that you will be there, no matter what—especially during the hard times. Make sure to be grateful to the people who stand by you, and do not take them for granted.

> You have likely faced great adversity, injustice, or loss in your life. Or you will. When you do, or when others do, stick together. Be kind. Love each other.

My sadness and pain didn't last long, however, because life goes on. Therefore, our work to protect life continued as well.

What Almost Stopped Me

"Success is the ability to go from failure to failure without losing enthusiasm."
—WINSTON CHURCHILL

When I declared Moms Across America—and essentially, myself—UNSTOPPABLE, I had no idea how much the universe would throw at me. I used the word "unstoppable" to encourage and support moms to keep going. Little did I know that there would be times when I felt not only stopped but also crushed. I have not been public about this, and I hesitate to be public about it now, because one cannot control the opinions that form in other people's minds. One cannot control their judgment and criticism. Pamm Larry, instigator of California's ballot initiative to label GMOs, helped me put things into perspective when she said, "What's the fastest way to get criticized? Do something."

Being UNSTOPPABLE does not always mean looking good, even though you are doing good. Sometimes it means your reputation is in the toilet, but you must keep going anyway. The right people to be on your team will come around. There were many times when I was so embarrassed by mistakes I had made that I wanted to just shut the whole thing down.

There was the time I trusted a source who said that the GMO salmon was not kosher because it contained eelpout fish genes and I posted a meme saying so. Eels are not kosher, but it turns out the eelpout is considered a fish even though it looks like an eel. Have you ever had the Jewish community condemn you? It's not fun.

There was the time when I used the phrase "tiny hydrogen molecules" when describing our Active H2 fundraiser molecular hydrogen product, when I meant to say that there are "tiny *amounts of* hydrogen molecules" in the tablet to infuse your water with hydrogen, compared to the huge amounts of hydrogen, say, in a blimp. The video went viral in the pro GMO community and the scientist I quoted got hammered with hate mail. Apparently, I am the stupidest person on the planet. I still get haters in my Facebook inbox telling me I'm an idiot.

There have been many internet vlogs and articles created to trash my reputation. One front group for the chemical companies decided that wasn't enough, however, so they spent untold amounts of money and a few years to make a documentary film to promote GMOs and discredit me and other food movement leaders. To hear what they had to say, I went to see the movie. I sat in a small art theater, albeit with only thirty other people, and felt the sting of the laughter around me when I spoke on the screen. The movie director had carefully edited what I said so that I would look foolish. It worked. Their manipulation of the footage likely had many people dismiss not only me but also moms in general as credible sources regarding the impact of GMOs. I was deeply sorry that I had allowed myself to be interviewed by these seemingly well-intentioned directors. I felt I let our moms down, and that they would be angry with me. Even worse, I feared that they would do exactly what the movie director's intended—they might lose hope and give up. Our moms are, of course, bigger than that. The ones I spoke to refused to watch the movie on principle. They gave me props for being a big enough threat to be in the company of Dr. Oz and Jeffrey Smith and cheered me on.

Many conventional farmers are not my biggest fans. They think I am out to take away their most valuable "tool"—glyphosate. They don't like that. Farmers have said they hope "that God will smite me dead." Shills have wished disease upon me. I have had many Facebook messaging conversations with farmers who seek me out to admonish me. Sometimes it's just a barrage of insults, but sometimes we can actually see something in common—we both want the farmers to be successful and healthy.

The worst situation for me—even more than being harassed—is when associates, organizations, or friends whom I respect shun me from their circles and exclude Moms Across America from events. Because it detracts from our effectiveness, the ultimate failure for me is being unable to work with others when I know we all have the same commitment. It's such a sad, unfortunate, and lost opportunity. Many nights I have lain awake, grieving the missed opportunities of working with other groups, blaming myself for being too pushy, or too naive, or too demanding . . . even if I do not know why they won't collaborate. They could simply be too busy! Yet it feels like a massive failure to me.

Then there were times when I don't feel I made a mistake—I just simply did not have the time or foresight to do certain things, like invite certain people to see test results weeks in advance of a press release. I often feel that if I don't do something right away—that is, if I wait for weeks for someone to weigh in—I won't get it done or the timing will be off. It will be too late to be of interest. So sometimes I rush things. Because of that people have judged me, thought me careless, selfish, or egotistical, and decided not to work with me. That hurt because it hurt our cause.

One night, I was up for over an hour, going back and forth with a person who was running a campaign for a GMO-free county, who was absolutely outraged because I had not posted about her campaign. She told me she went through two years of my posts to prove me wrong. Apparently, I had posted on one of the six Facebook pages I administer, but not our main Moms Across America page. I let her criticism give me anxiety. My heart seized up, and my chest hurt. I had trouble sleeping and I was just, well, sad.

I think the flip side of being passionate and driven is that I care deeply about what others think and I hurt deeply when I am thwarted. I am committed to everyone feeling empowered and for us to be effective and make progress . . . and when we don't, I feel like the worst kind of failure. At that point, I think that someone else is better suited to do this than me.

I am clear now, though, that all these other people are just doing what they are wont to do—expressing themselves and being committed to the cause in their own way. They didn't make me sad or stuck in a world of disempowerment instead of working on a new action—I did that.

What almost stopped me was *me,* my own thinking that I was messing up, or failing so much that I should stop, or that someone else would do a better job.

Some people think I am doing a great job—but the truth is, I have felt much more like a failure than a success. But that is what happens when one tries to take on a seemingly impossible task. I am working to transform the food industry and the health of America. And the world. That's a huge endeavor and one that is very far away from our current reality. But it's not impossible.

At Moms Across America, our motto is "Empowered Moms, Healthy Kids"—and that includes *all* moms and *all* kids. I have failed along the way because it is such a huge goal. There are hundreds of mom leaders who have volunteered, but I simply have not been able to connect with them. I have not returned calls, and many may feel I don't care and I am selfish or egotistical. Failure is bound to happen. I would be foolish not to expect it to happen. It is far more important for me to be failing at empowering moms to have healthy kids than it is for me to be winning at being right about not being the right one to do anything about it . . . and therefore taking no action.

The challenge lies not in the failures and the criticism, but in whether or not I choose to stop because of them. So I learn from my past actions. The next time I am trolled or criticized, I will take it less personally and learn from the experience. The next time I want a partner, rather than assuming that a person will work with me fifty-fifty as I would have in the past, because of my past mistakes I will ask what they can commit to. The next time I have a request to make of the attendees of an event I am organizing, I will make the request myself. I will simply learn from the failures in such a way that they become an essential part of my current success.

> The next time you are given an opportunity, do not stop yourself from saying "yes" because there was a "no" or difficulty in the past. Those past failures do not define you and do not determine your value or worth. They do not dictate your future or taint your past. Look for the opportunities and see if they align with your commitment. Then get clear about the expectations. When actions fail to happen, and they will, use this failure to your advantage. The most important thing is to not give up. Remember—regardless of what the universe throws your way, the only one that can stop you is you. You can simply choose to be UNSTOPPABLE.

PART FOUR

UNSTOPPABLE FUTURE

CHAPTER TWELVE
BELIEVE

"The future belongs to those who believe in the beauty of their dreams."
—ELEANOR ROOSEVELT

When I look to the future I want, I see a safe, uncompromised, healthy environment with an abundance and diversity of toxin-free organic crops, humanely treated animals, rich, clean soil, and plentiful, pure water. The future has a beautiful biodiversity—millions of butterflies, bees, fish, flora, and fauna that have my children marveling at the richness of nature and loving the great outdoors. The future I want is a world where our children are safe, healthy, prosperous, connected to nature, and have healthy relationships. This desire is universal.

While reading one of my childhood favorites, the iconic 1970s *Gnomes* book, to my then seven-year-old son Bronson who loved magical woodland creatures, we marveled at the bucolic scenery with rolling hills of lush, green bushes and fields. The gnomes had access to rabbit hair, flax, acorns, clean water, and plenty of nuts and berries. They lived in harmony with nature and they were appalled by the humans' habit of manipulation and exploitation of Earth's resources. As I read, "The salmon will always swim to spawn . . . the bees will always pollinate and make honey . . . and the butterflies will always flutter amongst the wildflowers . . . " my voice wavered. I realized suddenly that the fact they "always" would do it might not actually be true anymore.

I want my son to believe in gnomes because they are magical, compassionate, and live harmoniously with nature. I want him to be in that mystical forest in his imagination because our reality is so far from the gnomes' world. This is why we take our children camping in the outdoors for vacations, not to hotels in cities. I want them to see that some nature is still out there. I want my sons to have something to believe in.

To have them be a part of creating a future they can believe in, we have traveled cross-country, stayed at World Wide Opportunities on Organic Farms (WWOOF), and learned much about growing food. We have traveled partially or fully across the country four times, meeting inspiring, kind, and caring people who have given us faith in humanity. Back at home, we asked our landlord if we could stop using the gardener and take over our small, landscaped backyard, clear out the decorative plants, and grow food. He agreed. So, our new family project is growing food. When the seeds we have planted grow into food, that is magical to us. It's more work than just going to the grocery, but it is also much more fulfilling and is an important family bonding project. It gets us away from the TV and outside. We get inspiration for our garden when we see our neighbors' yards and when we travel. When we went on a nature hike in the nearby mountains we came across a miraculous swarm of ruby-colored ladybugs. The boys gently gathered some up and said they were going to bring them back to our garden, to protect our vegetables from aphids naturally. We are thrilled to harvest our tomatoes, potatoes, chives, parsley, cilantro, and lettuce without pesticides on them. My sons understand that many foods can be healing, remove toxins, and give them certain vitamins. I caught my son Ben having a late-night snack one night and asked him what he was eating. He replied, "An onion and garlic sandwich so that I feel better tomorrow for your birthday." He did feel better the next day. Nature is amazing. Our children can understand this if we just allow them to experience it firsthand.

More and more, people are learning the importance of growing our own food. Pamm Larry recently started the Good Food Brigade, highlighting people across the USA who are growing their own food. She is bringing back the concept of the victory gardens, which originated from war times when the government expected everyone to grow food in their backyards. In current times, because our food supply has become global, too many people are dependent on food from distant places. In times of climate change, chaos, and threats of war, growing food in our backyard and in our community is a wise local strategy that increases our homeland security. Creating a future where we are food secure and connected to local food growers strengthens America.

There is a huge surge of popularity in the homesteading movement that is exciting and inspiring. YouTube sensations like "Off Grid with Doug and Stacy" and John Kohler's "GrowYourGreens" have hundreds of thousands of viewers and are inspiring people to get out into nature, get their hands dirty with good bacteria, grow their own food, and be self-reliant. Taking actions that are self-reliant means not using toxic chemicals and working with nature. On our West Coast National Toxin Free Tour in 2017 we met supporters who were growing food forests, fish in aquaponics systems, raising chickens, fermenting foods, and making their own body care products. Just a few years ago, our social events were dominated by depressing conversations about health issues, the sorry state of our government, and food supply. Today, however, I find that we are excited to talk about herbal solutions, growing heirloom seeds, making household cleaners, and where to get good, local, organic, and seasonal fruits. We feel more connected to our friends and neighbors when we rely on ourselves and each other and share information and the fruit of our labor. People are realizing that self-reliance can lead to a celebration of community—a community not dictated by corporations and filtered by mass media, but one created by real, authentic, creative people who care about each other.

In the Beginning, There was Love . . .

> *"What lies behind you and what lies in front of you, pales in comparison to what lies inside of you."*
> —RALPH WALDO EMERSON

It was my son Ben's first day of life at our home and I held him in in my arms. He was tiny, pink, and delicate, wrapped in a blanket and still weighing almost nothing. Yet suddenly he was *everything* to me. As I gazed in awe at his sleeping face I said to my mother, "Isn't he amazing? Aren't *all* babies amazing?"

She touched my shoulder, looked at me with a smile in her eyes and said, "We all *still are*."

Wow.

In that moment, I saw how truly amazing my mother was and still is. I felt how much she loves not only me, but all people. I understood it was the same love I have for my son, and that this love is universal. We mothers love like that. Nothing will ever take away our amazement of our children. Babies and children are amazing . . . and when we grow up, we still are.

For a moment, however, I doubted my mother. I thought for sure, my newborn baby is much more amazing than I am. And that I am not as amazing now as I was when I was just a few days old, as if the amazing-ness sloughs off as we age. But as I allowed her love for me to soak in, and tears welled up in my eyes, I got that in her eyes, I am as amazing today as the day I was born. Just like my son does for me, I fill her with love and wonder. All she wants is for me to be happy and to be all that I can be in life.

I suddenly saw that I had a choice regarding how I saw myself. I could see myself through my own eyes as not amazing—or through her eyes, as unstoppably amazing. What if I saw myself from my mother's perspective? How much more fun would my life be? What if I saw other people—even the difficult ones—as amazing? What if all the people in the world saw themselves and others as amazing? We could accomplish so much more together!

What if a mother's love could transform the world?

I think it can. In fact, I know it can. I know deep in the marrow of my bones that the love of a mother can not only shift how our children see themselves, it can shift how they see the world—and their role in the world. Therefore, their actions in the world can come from that amazing-ness that we see them as having, and that amazing-ness will be expressed in the world. So, for a child, a mother's role is to not only to love and protect her children, it is also to be the one to see them as amazing, even when they don't see themselves that way. I wish for everyone to experience my mother's wisdom and understand how you, too, are truly amazing. It is a choice. Try it on. See yourself as amazing. See everyone you come in contact with or make a request of as amazing. If you do, you will suddenly see yourself as UNSTOPPABLE, and together we can transform the world.

UNSTOPPABLE Future—The Next Generation

> *"First they ignore you, then they laugh at you,
> then they fight you, then you win."*
> —MAHATMA GANDHI

When Gandhi stood before the British Parliament they said to him, "Little man, do you really think we are going to just hand India over to you?"

He nodded and said, "Yes."

He saw the British government as an entity that would eventually do the right thing. He saw the government (whether he liked it or not) as *great*. And doing so made him a great leader.

When we act *now*, change can happen *now*. I woke up on July 7, 2017, and realized it could be a historic day for our movement. It was the day that the California EPA's Office of Environmental Health Hazard Assessment (OEHHA) officially listed glyphosate on the California Prop 65 warning list as a carcinogen. The implications were huge. California has a population and economy larger than many countries around the world. Within a year, all companies with ten employees or more who manufacture products that expose humans to glyphosate above the "no significant risk level" (NSRL) will need to label that product with a warning such as, "This product contains a chemical which is known to cause cancer or reproductive harm." Now that glyphosate was on the Prop 65 carcinogen list, activists and city officials in California, the USA, and around the world had good and concrete reasons for discontinuing or banning the use of glyphosate.

> What if we see our policy makers and officials as great? What if we asked them to do the right thing? What could happen? A lot more than seeing them as wrong and assuming that they will do nothing.

OEHHA will first need to set a NSRL (which we hope will be zero, not the proposed 1,100 micrograms per day). Companies that make products that contain glyphosate will need to take into consideration bioaccumulation (the accumulation of a pesticide inside a human being).

If companies do not test for glyphosate and label their product with a Prop 65 warning, citizens can file a complaint. If the company is found to be violating the law to label, they can be fined up to $2,500 per day, per violation.

Depending on the final NSRL decided upon by OEHHA, food manufacturers may have to put labels on their food products in California that warn the consumer that they contain a chemical known to cause cancer. Without a doubt, products such as Roundup and other glyphosate-based herbicides will finally be labeled with a cancer warning. This is a dream come true for our movement. Short of removing the product from the market, it couldn't get any better than this.

We were excited for nearly a year with the thought that we had made huge strides. We thought the law would kick in and we would soon have warning labels on products. However, on February 27, 2018, one judge granted a preliminary injunction on the labeling aspect of the Prop 65 listing (but still left the chemical on the list) and temporarily halted manufacturers from being required to label their products. Although this was a huge setback for our movement, the fight is not over yet, and with strong lawyers and committed activists, we can still make major progress by citing glyphosate as being on the Prop 65 carcinogen list and the temporary no-labeling ruling. If there is one thing I have learned over the years, it is that the true marker of success has less to do with winning battles and much more to do with being UNSTOPPABLE. When we keep going, we win—no matter what the outcome. When we do not allow setbacks to stop us, but instead use them to propel us forward, we win. Regardless of court rulings, public opinion about toxic chemicals in our food supply is growing, and not reversing. Public opinion is such that the entire food movement is increasing the growing, buying, and eating of organic food. We are nearing the day when GMO and chemical farming will no longer be seen as viable, and faster than some think.

On that same day, July 7, 2017, I stood in line at the airport check-in, returning to California, the only state in our union to recognize the harmful effects of glyphosate, when I noticed a young man in his twenties with a T-shirt on that promoted cover crops. Cover crops are an eco-friendly method of planting a crop, such as clover, to crowd out and prevent other taller, more tenacious weeds, such as pigweed, from growing. Cover cropping can eliminate the use of herbicides completely and improve the quality of the soil. I was instantly excited. An ally! A sharp and informed young man! There was hope. I stepped over my duffel bag to move closer to him and asked him about his shirt. He said that he was a strategist for one of the largest food companies in the world. He had just come from a conference in Iowa where they were promoting cover crop methods to large food manufacturers. Trying to not appear like a five-year-old child who just got into Disneyland, I shared who I was and a little about our mission to raise awareness about GMOs and toxins. He nodded and said that all the big food companies such as Coca-Cola, Pepsi, and several others were in alignment to transition the agriculture industry to cover crop methods. I could have kissed him.

He was very excited to talk about cover cropping and the recent changes in the food system. I shared how I was so glad there was change happening. A year before, I had seen his food company's CEO speak at a conference where he tried convincing the foreign dignitaries to "not be anxious about local food security." In other words, let us—the USA—sell you our GMO food. Rest easy—we can feed the world. The young man agreed that the current farming system destroys our soil and poisons our water. I cited reports that the UK has only one generation left until their topsoil is depleted.

"If that," he added grimly. *He knew!*

We discussed farmers who say they have to spray because if they don't then they have to till—and that is worse. I said that I ask them to check out farmers Gabe Brown and Joel Salatin.

"Who are *killing it*," he said with a smile.

I was thrilled! Here was a strategist from one of the largest food conglomerates in the world *agreeing with me about the brilliance of regenerative, organic farmers Gabe Brown and Joel Salatin*. Agreeing with me about the solution! Progress! Less toxic chemicals and more sustainable farming, which protected the soil, the soil microbes, and our health. He went on to talk about how cover cropping was the solution. It was wonderful!

I brought up the fact that today was the day that the California EPA had officially listed glyphosate on the Prop 65 carcinogen list. "I am not surprised," he said, although his face did show concern. He asked about the implications of glyphosate being on the list.

I explained how if a child consumes conventional orange juice (which has tested positive for glyphosate) three times a week the manufacturer will have to add up the amount exposed over the lifetime of that child. If it exceeds 1,100 micrograms per day with bioaccumulation, the manufacturer will have to label that product with a warning. Wheat, bean, oat, and grain companies especially will have to do this. They won't want to however, so they will start to source growers who don't use glyphosate, and the solution to that is . . . "

"Cover cropping!" he and I said in unison.

"This is the solution," he said with an authentically warm smile. I told him that we would really like to celebrate the leadership of his company. I acknowledged that they were one of the first big companies to begin sourcing GMO-free products because the consumers wanted them, and we were thrilled about their responsiveness.

This conversation made me feel more hopeful than I had been in years. Here was a young man who knew what the world needed. Here was a youth, taking a stand for a healthy world. A man much like my sons are growing up to be and who is already in a position to influence the most powerful companies in the world. I asked him if his background was in farming, and he said, "No, in economics." *Of course,* I thought. *It all comes down to money.* But then I realized that it was perfect—economists were getting that GMO chemical farming was not economically viable and that it was not working!

I was overwhelmed with joy.

I will not wait to celebrate the success our movement has made. The success is here. The youth get it. They are making a difference. We are all amazing and UNSTOPPABLE. The food industry, whether it likes it or not, is being transformed.

CONCLUSION

Over the years of being involved in this frustrating and infuriating—yet also fascinating and empowering—food movement, I have met people of all ages and backgrounds like this young man. All generations want this toxic food system to be fixed *now*. When my family and I traveled cross-country in 2015 and again on our National Toxin Free Tour in 2016 and 2017 (the subject of our documentary *Communities Rising*), we met people in big corporations, small businesses, schools, churches, health care, campgrounds, organic farms, and small towns. All of them wanted the same things—safe food, clean water, and healthy families. It is right and fair that they want these things. No one has the right to take these things from us. We have the right to choose. We have the right to not be poisoned. Beyond rights, we strive to thrive—and will continue to do so.

Together, we are going beyond the current circumstances and we are creating a future to be proud of—one of health, freedom, and justice. We are recovering our children and our health. We are restoring the potential of our children and the future of our country. Every day, we have a choice. Every day, we have an opportunity to teach our children what love is . . . which means taking actions to create a future that we can be proud of . . . safe, free, healthy, and thriving. They are listening to us and they are watching.

My son, Ben, was the first in our family to talk about GMOs and pesticides in food when he made a presentation in fourth grade titled "Healthy Happy Students." Now, at fifteen, he says, "This problem of GMOs and pesticides in our food needs to be fixed now. The greatest threat is not the problem, however. It is the idea that someone else will do something about it."

He has faith however, that "our generation will fix it, because we are all directly affected by GMOs and pesticides." He states that, "Information spreads and cannot be stopped."

We cannot be stopped. The time is now . . . and the next generation has our back. Together, we've got this.

> The pathway to triumph, empowerment, and celebration of community is a rewarding and enriching process:
>
> 1. Get present to how much you love your family. Love them and listen to them.
>
> 2. Educate yourself and be willing to face the difficult truths.
>
> 3. Get connected with a diverse community, learn from others, and ask questions.
>
> 4. Take action. Do one thing a day. Detox, share information, make calls or send emails, buy organic, and grow your own food. Step into leadership and host an event or invite people to join your local parade. Create the future you want.
>
> 5. Acknowledge and celebrate progress, both your own and other people's. Share the wins, celebrate your community, and see the joy in the triumphs of the human spirit.

The food industry may be broken and bought but the people of America and the world are not. We are creative, courageous, and are making a huge contribution to each other's lives by speaking up and taking action. We will not stop! We will not give up! The love for our families and for freedom will never end!

RESOURCES

Website Sources
Alter Trade Japan: www.altertrade.co.jp/english/01/01_02_e.html
Camp of the Sacred Stones: http://sacredstonecamp.org/
Center for Food Safety: https://www.centerforfoodsafety.org/
Cultured Food Life (Donna Schwenk's website): www.culturedfoodlife.com
Earth Day Network: www.earthday.org
Factory Farming Awareness Coalition: http://www.ffacoalition.org/
Food Babe: www.foodbabe.com
GMO Free PA Lancaster County: https://www.facebook.com/GMOFreePALancaster/
John Kohler: https://www.youtube.com/user/growingyourgreens
Landmark: www.landmarkworldwide.com
March Against Monsanto: www.march-against-monsanto.com
Moms Across America: www.momsacrossamerica.org
National Health Freedom Coalition: https://nationalhealthfreedom.org
Non-Toxic Communities: https://nontoxiccommunities.com/
Off Grid with Doug and Stacy: https://www.youtube.com/watch?v=c1FBd4ihp_c
Organic Consumers Association: https://www.organicconsumers.org/
People for the Ethical Treatment of Animals (PETA): https://www.peta.org
Robyn O'Brien: www.robynobrien.com
Séralini and team: http://www.criigen.org/
Sierra Club: www.sierraclub.org
The Cornucopia Institute: https://www.cornucopia.org/
The Good Food Brigade: www.goodfoodbrigade.org
The Green Co-Op Union (Japan): www.greencoop.or.jp
The Shaka Movement: www.mauigmomoratoriumnews.org
The Thinking Moms' Revolution: http://thinkingmomsrevolution.com
The Truth About Vaccines: https://go.thetruthaboutvaccines.com
Vaccine Information Center: www.nvic.org
Vaccines Revealed: www.vaccinesrevealed.com
Wheat Belly blog http://www.wheatbellyblog.com/2012/08/down-and-out-wheat-addiction/

GMO News Sites
Earth Open Source: www.earthopensource.org
GMO Evidence: www.gmoevidence.com
 GMO Free USA: www.gmofreeusa.comSustainable Pulse:
GMWatch: www.GMwatch.com
 Sustainable Pulse: www.sustainablepulse.com
The Non-GMO Project Verified: www.nongmoproject.org

Films

"Alice Gleason from Uganda" (video) http://www.momsacrosstheworld.com/videos
BOUGHT: www.youtube.com/watch?v=CSAhXeB_jzA
Communities Rising: www.youtube.com/watch?v=DHa-Om3jWas&t=5s
Consumed: www.consumedthemovie.com/
Food, Inc.: www.netflix.com/title/70108783
Genetic Roulette: www.responsibletechnology.org
GMO OMG: www.gmofilm.com/
"How Wolves Change Rivers" (video) https://www.youtube.com/watch?v=ysa5OBhXz-Q
List of GMO and food movies http://www.momsacrossamerica.com/movies_about_gmos
MODIFIED: www.indiegogo.com/projects/modified-food#/
Poisoned Fields: Glyphosate, the Underrated Risk? https://www.youtube.com/watch?v=XDyI10Z8aH0&t=307s
SEED: The Untold Story: www.seedthemovie.com/
The Future of Food: www.thefutureoffood.com/
"The Secrets of Sugar" (video from the Canadian Broadcasting Channel) https://www.youtube.com/watch?v=xDaYa0AB8TQ
Vaxxed: From Cover-Up to Catastrophe: http://vaxxedthemovie.com/
What's With Wheat?: https://whatswithwheat.com/

Books

Allen, Will. *The War on Bugs*. Chelsea Green Publishing, 2007.
Campbell-McBride, Natasha. *Gut and Psychology Syndrome: Natural Treatment for Autism, Dyspraxia, A.D.D., Dyslexia, A.D.H.D., Depression, Schizophrenia*. Medinform Publishing, 2010.
Diamandis, Peter H. *Bold: How to Go Big, Create Wealth, and Impact the World*. Simon & Schuster, 2015.
Drucker, Steven. *Altered Genes, Twisted Truth: How the Venture to Genetically Engineer Our Food Has Subverted Science, Corrupted Government, and Systematically Deceived the Public*. Clear River Press, 2015.
Gates, Donna. *The Body Ecology Diet: Recovering Your Health and Rebuilding Your Immunity*. Hay House, 2011.
Gillam, Carey. *Whitewash: The Story of a Weed Killer, Cancer, and the Corruption of Science*. Island Press, 2017.
Hari, Vani. *The Food Babe Way: Break Free from the Hidden Toxins in Your Food and Lose Weight, Look Years, and Get Healthy in Just 21 Days!*. Little, Brown and Company, 2015.
Hauter, Wynona. *Foodopoly: The Battle over the Future of Food and Farming in America*. The New Press, 2012.
Humphries, Suzanne. *Dissolving Illusions: Disease, Vaccines, and the Forgotten History*. CreateSpace Independent Publishing, 2014.
Kahn, Joel. *The Whole Heart Solution: Halt Heart Disease Now with the Best Alternative and Traditional Medicine*. Reader's Digest, 2014.
Keyes, April Scott. *GMO-Free Child: A Parent's Guide to Dietary Cleanup of Genetically Modified Organisms*. First Books, 2016.
Mitra, Tony. *Poisoned Foods of North America: Guide to Navigating the Glyphosate Mine Field in Our Food Web*. Independently published, 2017.
O'Brien, Robyn. *The Unhealthy Truth: One Mother's Shocking Investigation into the Dangers of*

America's Food Supply—and What Every Family Can Do to Protect Itself. Harmony Books, 2010.

Patterson, Susan. *15 Minute Healthy, Organic Meals for Less than $10 a Day.* Through God's Grace Publishing, 2014.

Perro, Michelle. *What's Making Our Children Sick?: How Industrial Food Is Causing an Epidemic of Chronic Illness, and What Parents (and Doctors) Can Do about It.* Chelsea Green Publishing, 2017.

Rodale, Maria. *The Organic Manifesto: How Organic Food Can Heal Our Planet, Feed the World, and Keep Us Safe.* Rodale Books, 2011.

Segerston, Alissa and Malterre, Tom. *The Elimination Diet: Discover the Foods That Are Making You Sick and Tired—and Feel Better Fast* by. Grand Central Life & Style, 2016.

Smith, Jeffrey M. *Seeds of Destruction: Exposing Industry and Government Lies about the Safety of the Genetically Engineered Foods You're Eating.* Yes! Books, 2003.

Vallianatos, Evaggelos. *Poison Spring: The Secret History of Pollution and the FDA.* Bloomsbury Press, 2014.

Wood, Robert. *Food Allergies for Dummies.* John Wiley and Sons Ltd., 2007.

We wish to express the deepest gratitude to the sponsors, foundations, and individuals who support Moms Across America. Our current sponsors are shown on our website at www.momsacrossamerica.org.

NOTES

Part One: UNSTOPPABLE Love

Chapter One: Love in Action
The Erosion of Health and Mom Power
1. Cancer rates: 2007 Surveillance Epidemiology and End Results (SEER) program at the National Cancer Institute (NCI), Medscape: https://www.medscape.com/viewarticle/551998.
2. Mental Illness: National Alliance on Mental Illness; "Mental Health By The Numbers" https://www.nami.org/learn-more/mental-health-by-the-numbers.
3. Liver disease: "Do You Have Liver Damage?" by Dr. Manny https://www.askdrmanny.com/do-you-have-liver-damage/.

Put the Oxygen Mask on Yourself First . . .
4. Gluten Intolerance: "3 Reasons Gluten Intolerance May Be More Serious Than Celiac Disease," by Chris Kresser, June 16, 2015, https://chriskresser.com/3-reasons-gluten-intolerance-may-be-more-serious-than-celiac-disease/.

Chapter Two: Learning the Truth about GMOs
Understanding the Problem
1. GMOs: "Genetically Engineered Crops, Glyphosate and the Deterioration of Health in the United States," by Nancy L. Swanson, Andre Leu, Jon Abrahamson, and Bradley Wallet.
2. "GMOs: Autism and Altered Intestinal Bacteria Associated with High Intake of GMO-Foods and Exposure to Weed-Killer, Glyphosate-Elevated Urinary Glyphosate and Clostridia Metabolites with Altered Dopamine Metabolism in Triplets with Autistic Spectrum Disorder or Suspected Seizure Disorder: A Case Study," by William Shaw, Ph.D.
3. Birth Defects: "Glyphosate-Based Herbicides Produce Teratogenic Effects on Vertebrates by Impairing Retinoic Acid Signaling," by Alejandra Paganelli, Victoria Gnazzo, Helena Acosta, Silvia L. López, and Andrés E. Carrasco, *Chemical Research in Toxicology*, 2010.
4. Bt Toxin: "3.8 Myth: GM Bt Insecticidal Crops Only Harm Insects and Are Harmless to Animals and People. Truth: GM Bt Insecticidal Crops Pose Hazards to People and Animals That Eat Them" (part of "GMO Myths & Truths"), http://earthopensource.org/gmomythsandtruths/sample-page/3-health-hazards-gm-foods/3-8-myth-gm-bt-insecticidal-crops-harm-insects-harmless-animals-people/.
5. GMOs: "An integrated multi-omics analysis of the NK603 Roundup-tolerant GM maize reveals metabolism disturbances caused by the transformation process." by Robin Mesnage, Sarah Z. Agapito-Tenfen, Vinicius Vilperte, George Renney, Malcolm Ward, Gilles-Éric Séralini, Rubens O. Nodari, and Michael N. Antoniou, *Scientific Reports* volume 6, Article number: 37855 (2016) doi:10.1038/srep37855 https://www.nature.com/articles/srep37855.
6. Glyphosate: "Glyphosate Fact Sheet," *Journal of Pesticide Reform*.

7. Glyphosate: "Long term toxicity of a Roundup herbicide and a Roundup-tolerant genetically modified maize," by Gilles-Éric Séralini, Emilie Clair, Robin Mesnage, Steve Gress, Nicolas Defarge, Manuela Malatesta, and Didier Hennequin. June 24, 2014, *Environmental Sciences Europe* Bridging Science and Regulation at the Regional and European Level201426:1 https://doi.org/10.1186/s12302-014-0014-5.
8. https://enveurope.springeropen.com/articles/10.1186/s12302-014-0014-5
9. GMOs: "The Shikimate Pathway, the Microbiome, and Disease: Health Effects of GMOs on Humans," by Jeanne D'Brant, Associate Professor of Biology & Allied Health, State University of NY. http://teca.fao.org/sites/default/files/comments/files/GMO%2CShikimate_pathway_gut_flora_and_health.pdf.
10. Nano Technology: http://www.foodpackagingforum.org/.
11. Synthetic Biology: Friends of the Earth—Synthetic Biology GMOs 2.0 Guide. https://foe.org/resources/gmos-2-0-synthetic-biology-guide/.
12. CRISPR Technology: "CRISPR Gene-Editing Can Cause Hundreds of Unexpected Mutations," BEC Crew, Science Alert, May 30, 2017, https://www.sciencealert.com/turns-out-crispr-gene-editing-can-cause-hundreds-of-unexpected-mutations.
13. Pesticides and Depression: "Farmer Suicide Rates Higher than Veterans" Newsweek magazine, by Max Kutner, June 13, 2016, magazine.http://www.newsweek.com/farmer-suicide-rate-higher-veterans-479823.
14. Gut bacteria and glyphosate: "Effects of Roundup and Glyphosate on Three Food Microorganisms: Geotrichum candidum, Lactococcus lactis subsp. cremoris and Lactobacillus delbrueckii subsp. Bulgaricus," by Emilie Clair, Laura Linn, Carine Travert, Caroline Amiel, and Gilles-Éric Séralini, Current Microbiology. May 2012, Vol. 64 Issue 5, p486-491.
15. Goats and GMO feed: "Genetically modified soybean in a goat diet: Influence on kid performance," by R. Tudiscoa, S. Calabròa, M.I. Cutrignellia, G. Moniellob, M. Grossia, V. Mastellonea, P. Lombardia, M.E. Peroa, and F. Infascelli. Science Direct, Small Ruminant Research, Volume 126, Supplement 1, May 2015, Pages 67-7 https://doi.org/10.1016/j.smallrumres.2015.01.023.
16. Hamsters, GMOs, and Sterility: "Genetically Modified Soy Linked to Sterility, Infant Mortality in Hamsters," by Jeffrey M. Smith, May 25, 2011, http://www.responsibletechnology.org/blog/18.
17. Pigs and GMOs: "Biological impact of feeding rats with a genetically modified-based diet," by Hanaa Oraby, Mahrousa Kandil, Nermeen Shaffie, and Inas Ghaly, Cell Biology Department, Genetic Engineering and Biotechnology Division, National Research Center, Cairo, Egypt, Turkish Journal of Biology January 2015 Volume 39(2):1-11.
18. Paper on Glyphosate: "Glyphosate pathways to modern diseases V: Amino acid analogue of glycine in diverse proteins," by Anthony Samsel and Stephanie Seneff, Journal of Biological Physics and Chemistry Volume 16(June):9-46 · June 2016.
19. Glyphosate: "Glyphosate's Suppression of Cytochrome P450 Enzymes and Amino Acid Biosynthesis by the Gut Microbiome: Pathways to Modern Diseases," by Anthony Samsel and Stephanie Seneff, *Entropy* 2013, *15*(4), 1416-1463.
20. Glyphosate and Gut Bacteria: "The Effect of Glyphosate on Potential Pathogens and Beneficial Members of Poultry Microbiota In Vitro," by Awad A. Shehata, Wieland Schrodl, Alaa. A. Aldin, Hafez M. Hafez, and Monika Kruger, Curr Microbiol. 2013 Apr;66(4):350-8.
21. Antibiotic Resistance and Glyphosate: "Sublethal Exposure to Commercial Formulations of the Herbicides Dicamba, 2,4-Dichlorophenoxyacetic Acid, and Glyphosate Cause Changes in Antibiotic Susceptibility in Escherichia coli and Salmonella enterica serovar Typhimurium," by Brigitta Kurenbacha, Delphine Marjoshia, Carlos F. Amábile-Cuevasb, Gayle C. Fergusonc, William

Godsoed, Paddy Gibsona, and Jack A. Heinemann. MBio, March 2014.
22. GMOs and Glyphosate: "GMO Crop Pathogen and Infertility—Glyphosate Pesticide Dangers," Presentation given by Dr. Huber in Kauai, September 2015, https://www.youtube.com/watch?v=-jkQzaCaFsY.
23. Glyphosate: Special Release: GLYPHOSATE (A PAN AP Factsheet), http://archive.panap.net/en/p/post/pesticides-info-database/1378.
24. Glyphosate: "The Effect of Glyphosate on Potential Pathogens and Beneficial Members of Poultry Microbiota In Vitro," by Awad A. Shehata, Wieland Schrodl, Alaa. A. Aldin, Hafez M. Hafez, and Monika Kruger, Curr Microbiol. 2013 Apr;66(4):350-8. doi: 10.1007/s00284-012-0277-2. Epub 2012 Dec 9.
25. Glyphosate: "Elevated Urinary Glyphosate and Clostridia Metabolites With Altered Dopamine Metabolism in Triplets With Autistic Spectrum Disorder or Suspected Seizure Disorder: A Case Study," by William Shaw, Ph.D, Integr Med (Encinitas). 2017 Feb;16(1):50-57.
26. Glyphosate: "Glyphosate-based herbicides are toxic and endocrine disruptors in human cell lines," by Céline Gasnier, Coralie Dumont, Nora Benachour, Emilie Clair, Marie-Christine Chagnon, and Gilles-Éric Séralini, Toxicology. 2009 Aug 21;262(3):184-91. doi: 10.1016/j.tox.2009.06.006. Epub 2009 Jun 17.
27. Glyphosate: "Endocrine disruption and cytotoxicity of glyphosate and roundup in human JAr cells in vitro," by Fiona Young, Dao Ho, Danielle Glynn, and Vicki Edwards. OAT, DOI: 10.15761/IPTG.1000114.
28. Glyphosate: "Glyphosate-based herbicides Produce Teratogenic Effects on Vertebrates by Impairing Retinoic Acid Signaling," by Alejandra Paganelli, Victoria Gnazzo, Helena Acost, Silvia L. Lopez, and Andre Carrasco, Chem Res Toxicol. 2010 Oct 18;23(10):1586-95. doi: 10.1021/tx1001749. Epub 2010 Aug 9.
29. Glyphosate: "Roundup disrupts male reproductive functions by triggering calcium-mediated cell death in rat testis and Sertoli cells," by Vera Lúciade, Liz Oliveira Cavalli, Daiane Cattani, Carla Elise Heinz Rieg, Paula Pierozan, Leila Zanatta, Eduardo Benedetti Parisotto, Danilo Wilhelm Filho, Fátima Regina Mena Barreto Silva, Regina Pessoa-Pureur, and Ariane Zamoner, Free Radic Biol Med. 2013 Dec;65:335-46. doi: 10.1016/j.freeradbiomed.2013.06.043. Epub 2013 Jun 29.
30. Glyphosate: "Roundup disrupts male reproductive functions by triggering calcium-mediated cell death in rat testis and Sertoli cells," by Vera Lúcia de Liz Oliveira Cavalli, Daiane Cattani, Carla Elise Heinz Rieg, Paula Pierozan , Leila Zanatta, Eduardo Benedetti Parisotto, Danilo Wilhelm Filho, Fátima Regina Mena Barreto Silva, Regina Pessoa-Pureur, Ariane Zamoner, Elsevier, June 2013.
31. Glyphosate: "Perinatal exposure to glyphosate-based herbicide alters the thyrotrophic axis and causes thyroid hormone homeostasis imbalance in male rats," by Janaina Senade, Souzaa Marina, Malta LetroKizysa, Rodrigo Rodriguesda Conceiçãoa, Gabriel Glebockia, Renata Marino Romanob, Tania Maria Ortiga Carvalhoc, Gisele Giannoccoa, Ismael Dale, Cotrim Guerreiroda, Silvad Magnus, Regios Diasda, Silvaa Marco Aurélio Romanob, and Maria Izabel Chiamoleraa, Toxicology, Volume 377, 15 February 2017, Pages 25-37.
32. Autism correlation to glyphosate use: "What if the consumption of GMO crops or animals eating GMO crops were related to rapid rise of these chronic diseases?" by Nancy Swanson, Ph.D.http://www.biobased.us/Nancy%20Swanson%20What%20if%20GMO.html.
33. Co-Formulants: "Co-Formulants in Glyphosate-Based Herbicides Disrupt Aromatase Activity in Human Cells below Toxic Levels," by Nicolas Defarge, Eszter Takács, Verónica Laura Lozano, Robin Mesnage, Joël Spiroux de Vendômois, Gilles-Éric Séralini, and András Székács, Int J Environ Res Public Health. 2016 Feb 26;13(3). pii: E264. doi: 10.3390/ijerph13030264.
34. American Mind Melt: "Mechanisms underlying the neurotoxicity induced by glyphosate-based

herbicide in immature rat hippocampus: Involvement of glutamate excitotoxicity," by Daiane Cattani, Vera Lúcia de Liz Oliveira Cavalli, Carla Elise Heinz Rieg, Juliana Tonietto Domingues, Tharine Dal-Cim, Carla Inês Tasca, Fátima Regina Mena Barreto Silva, and Ariane Zamoner, Toxicology. 2014 Jun 5;320:34-45. doi: 10.1016/j.tox.2014.03.001. Epub 2014 Mar 15.
35. Glyphosate in Vaccines: "Glyphosate Found in Childhood Vaccines" by Zen Honeycutt, Moms Across America, September 6, 2016, https://www.momsacrossamerica.com/glyphosate_found_in_childhood_vaccines.
36. Séralini's study on Roundup and Rats: "Republished study: Long term toxicity of a Roundup herbicide and a Roundup-tolerant genetically modified maize," by Séralini, G. E., et al., https://enveurope.springeropen.com/articles/10.1186/s12302-014-0014-5.
37. Rodent Diets: "Laboratory Rodent Diets Contain Toxic Levels of Environmental Contaminants: Implications for Regulatory Tests," by Robin Mesnage, Nicolas Defarge, Louis-Marie Rocque, Joël Spiroux de Vendômois, and Gilles-Éric Séralini.
38. Glyphosate and Cancer: "Glyphosate induces human breast cancer cells growth via estrogen receptors," by Thongprakaisang S, Thiantanawat A, Rangkadilok N, Suriyo T, and Satayavivad J, Food Chem Toxicol. 2013 Sep;59:129-36. doi: 10.1016/j.fct.2013.05.057. Epub June 1, 2013.
39. Glyphosate: "Glyphosate-based herbicides are toxic and endocrine disruptors in human cell lines," by Céline Gasnier, Coralie Dumont, Nora Benachour, Emilie Clair, Marie-Christine Chagnon, and Gilles-Éric Séralini, Toxicology. 2009 Aug 21;262(3):184-91. doi: 10.1016/j.tox.2009.06.006. Epub 2009 Jun 17.
40. GMOs: "The Biggest GMO Myths, Busted. Genetic modification isn't all it's cracked up to be. For starters, it's causing us to use more chemical pesticides," by Leah Zerb, Rodale Institute. https://www.rodalesorganiclife.com/food/gmo-myths.
41. Glyphosate: "Updated Screening Level Usage Analysis (SLUA) Report for Glyphosate," United States Environmental Protection Agency, October 22, 2015.
42. Human exposure to glyphosate has increased 500 percent: "Exposure to Glyphosate, Chemical Found in Weed Killers, Increased Over 23 Years," by Yadira Galindo UC San Diego Health https://health.ucsd.edu/news/releases/Pages/2017-10-24-exposure-to-glyphosate-chemical-found-in-weed-killer-increased-over-23-years.aspx.
43. Glyphosate: "EPA increase of glyphosate residues on food crops 2013," Environmental Protection Agency. Originally published by The Washington Times, Communities, July 5, 2013.
44. Glyphosate: "Potential toxic effects of glyphosate and its commercial formulations below regulatory limits," by R. Mesange, N. Defarge, J. Spiroux de Vendômois, and G. E. Séralini, Food and Chemical Toxicology, Volume 84, October 2015, Pages 133-153.
45. Glyphosate: "Glyphosate Sprayed on GMO Crops Linked to Lake Erie's Toxic Algae Bloom," by Lorraine Chow, Ecowatch, July 5, 2016, https://www.ecowatch.com/glyphosate-sprayed-on-gmo-crops-linked-to-lake-eries-toxic-algae-bloom-1906543478.html.
46. Semen quality in China drastic decline: "Decline in semen quality among 30,636 young Chinese men from 2001 to 2015," by Chuan Huang, Ph.D, et al., Institute of Reproductive and Stem Cell Engineering, Fertil Steril. 2017 Jan;107(1):83-88.e2. doi: 10.1016/j.fertnstert.2016.09.035. Epub 2016 Oct 25.
47. US, UK, and Australian sperm quality rates: "Temporal trends in sperm count: a systematic review and meta-regression analysis," by Hagai Levine, Niels Jørgensen, Anderson Martino Andrade, Jaime Mendiola, Dan Weksler-Derri, Irina Mindlis, Rachel Pinotti, and Shanna H. Swan, *Human Reproduction Update*, Volume 23, Issue 6, 1 November 2017, Pages 646–659, https://doi.org/10.1093/humupd/dmx022.
48. Glyphosate: "A critical review of glyphosate findings in human urine samples and comparison with the exposure of operators and consumers," by Lars Niemann, Christian Sieke Rudolf, and

Pfeil Roland Solecki, Journal für Verbraucherschutz und Lebensmittelsicherheit, March 2015, Volume 10, Issue 1, pp 3–12.
49. Glyphosate: "Glyphosate, pathways to modern diseases II: Celiac sprue and gluten intolerance," by Anthony Samsel and Stephanie Seneff, *Interdisciplinary Toxicology*, Interdiscip Toxicol. 2013 Dec;6(4):159-84. doi: 10.2478/intox-2013-0026.
50. Nutrition: "Nutritional Quality of Organic Versus Conventional Fruits, Vegetables, and Grains," by Virginia Worthington, *Journal of Alternative and Complementary Medicine*, July 2004.

Chapter Three: Learning the Truth about Glyphosate
Glyphosate in My Son
1. Glyphosate: US Geological Survey (USGS) Glyphosate found in streams: https://toxics.usgs.gov/highlights/glyphosate02.html.

Testing for Glyphosate
2. Glyphosate: "Toxic Breast Milk?" by Florence Williams, The New York Times, January 9, 2005.
3. Glyphosate: "Glyphosate Testing Full Report: Findings in American Mothers' Breast Milk, Urine and Water," by Zen Honeycutt, Moms Across America and Henry Rowlands, Sustainable Pulse, April 7, 2014.
4. EPA mission: https://www.epa.gov/aboutepa/our-mission-and-what-we-do.
5. EPA: "The EPA has only banned these 9 chemicals—out of thousands," by Rebecca Harrington, February 10, 2016.
6. Endocrine disruptors: "42-billion-dollar loss from endocrine disruptors—Exposure to endocrine-disrupting chemicals in the USA: a population-based disease burden and cost analysis."Attina, Hauser, Sathyanarayana, Hunt, Bourguignon, Myers, DiGangi, Zoeller, Trasande, Lancet Diabetes Endocrinol. 2016 Dec;4(12):996-1003. doi: 10.1016/S2213-8587(16)30275-3. Epub 2016 Oct 17.
7. Monsanto: "How Monsanto Captured the EPA (And Twisted Science) To Keep Glyphosate on the Market. Since 1973, Monsanto has cited dubious science, like tests on the uteri of male mice, and the EPA has let much of it slide," by Valeria Brown and Elizabeth Grossman, November 2017.
8. Glyphosate: "3 Studies Proving Toxic Glyphosate in Urine, Bloodstream and Breast milk," by Mike Barrett Natural Society, May 4, 2014.
9. "The effect of metabolites and impurities of glyphosate on human erythrocytes (in vitro)." Pestic Biochem Physiol. 2014 Feb; 109:34-43. doi: 10.1016/j.pestbp.2014.01.003. Epub 2014 Jan 25.
10. Glyphosate: "Glyphosate Found in Feeding Tube Liquid Given to Children with Cancer" by Zen Honeycutt, Moms Across America, January 2015 https://www.momsacrossamerica.com/glyphosate_found_in_feeding_tube_liquid.
11. Inflammation: "8 Food Ingredients That Can Cause Inflammation," Arthritis Foundation. https://www.arthritis.org/living-with-arthritis/arthritis-diet/foods-to-avoid-limit/food-ingredients-and-inflammation.php.
12. Glyphosate: "Glyphosate induces cardiovascular toxicity in Danio rerio," by Nicole M. Roy, Jeremy Ochs, Ewelina Zambrzycka, and Ariann Anderson, Environ Toxicol Pharmacol. 2016 Sep;46:292-300. doi: 10.1016/j.etap.2016.08.010. Epub 2016 Aug 11.
13. Glyphosate: "World Health Organization: Glyphosate is a Probable Carcinogen," Kathryn Z Guyton, Dana Loomis, Yann Grosse, Fatiha El Ghissassi, Lamia Benbrahim-Tallaa, Neela Guha, Chiara Scoccianti, Heidi Mattock, Kurt Straif, on behalf of the International Agency for Research on Cancer Monograph Working Group, IARC, Lyon, France, GMOevidence.com https://www.gmoevidence.com/world-health-organization-glyphosate-is-a-probable-human-carcinogen/.

14. Paper by Samsel and Seneff Showing Glyphosate and Cancer Causing Properties Known By EPA since 1983: "Glyphosate, pathways to modern diseases IV: cancer and related pathologies," by Anthony Samsel and Stephanie Seneff, Journal of Biological Physics and Chemistry 15(3):121-159 January 2015.
15. Glyphosate: "Study: Glyphosate Doubles Risk of Lymphoma," by Emily Cassidy, Research Analyst, By Emily Cassidy, Environmental Working Group, Friday, May 23, 2014.https://www.ewg.org/agmag/2014/05/study-glyphosate-doubles-risk-lymphoma#.WrRzLZPwZ-U.
16. Roundup: "Monsanto's Roundup Under Fire in CA," by Zen Honeycutt, Moms Across America, June 10, 2017, https://www.momsacrossamerica.com/monsanto_s_roundup_under_fire_in_ca.
17. Glyphosate: "Glyphosate and Cancer Risks Frequently Asked Questions," Center for Food Safety, May 2015 https://www.centerforfoodsafety.org/fact-sheets/3920/glyphosate-and-cancer-risk-frequently-asked-questions.
18. GMOs: "Kellogg's Fruit Loops Test Positive for GMOs and Weed killer," 2013.https://gmofreeusa.org/food-testing/kelloggs/kelloggs-froot-loops/
19. Glyphosate: "ANH Releases Study of Glyphosate in Breakfast Foods," by ANH-USA April 19, 2016, http://www.anh-usa.org/anh-releases-study-of-glyphosate-in-breakfast-foods/.
20. Glyphosate: "FDA Finds Monsanto's Weed Killer in US Honey," by Carey Gillam, HuffPost, September 16, 2017, https://www.huffingtonpost.com/carey-gillam/fda-finds-monsantos-weed_b_12008680.html.
21. Glyphosate: "FDA Test Confirm Glyphosate in Oatmeal, Baby Food Contains Residues of Monsanto Weedkiller," by Carey Gillam, HuffPost December 6, 2017, https://www.huffingtonpost.com/carey-gillam/fda-tests-confirm-oatmeal_b_12252824.html.
22. Glyphosate: "Argentinian Study: Tampons, Sanitary Pads and Sterile Gauze Contaminated with Probable Carcinogen Glyphosate," Henry Rowlands, The Detox Project, October 2015, https://detoxproject.org/argentinian-study-tampons-sanitary-pads-and-sterile-gauze-contaminated-with-probable-carcinogen-glyphosate/.
23. Glyphosate: "Monsanto's Glyphosate Found in California Wine," by Zen Honeycutt, ECO Watch March 27, 2016, https://www.ecowatch.com/monsantos-glyphosate-found-in-california-wines-even-wines-made-with-or-1882199552.html.
24. Irritable Bowel Syndrome: "Canadian Digestive Health Foundation Public Impact Series 3: Irritable bowel syndrome in Canada. Incidence, prevalence, and direct and indirect economic impact," by Richard N Fedorak, MD, et al., Can J Gastroenterol. 2012 May; 26(5): 252–256.
25. Glyphosate: "Glyphosate Found in All 5 Major Orange Juice Brands," by Zen Honeycutt, October 11, 2017, https://www.momsacrossamerica.com/all_top_5_orange_juice_brands_positive_for_weedkiller.
26. Copper used on Citrus: "Copper Fungicides for Citrus Trees," by Victoria Lee Blackstone, SF Gate, http://homeguides.sfgate.com/copper-fungicides-citrus-trees-49339.html.
27. Copper is effective spermicide: "One Thing No One Tells You About the Copper IUD," by Jr. Thorpe, February 29, 2016, https://www.bustle.com/articles/144818-the-one-thing-nobody-tells-you-about-the-copper-iud.
28. Disturbing Toxin Test Results: "Some 'Healthy' Foods are Poisoning Us," by Zen Honeycutt, May 5, 2017, https://www.momsacrossamerica.com/some_healthy_foods_are_poisoning_us

Health in America Today

29. Health: "New Health Rankings: Of 17 Nations, US Is Dead Last," by Grace Rubenstein, *The Atlantic,* January 10, 2017.
30. Health: "1 out of 2 children have a chronic illness," by Maria Rickert Hong, Kid's Health.

31. Diabetes: "New CDC report: More than 100 million Americans have diabetes or prediabetes," July 18, 2017. https://www.cdc.gov/media/releases/2017/p0718-diabetes-report.html.
32. Cancer: "Cancer Strikes 1 in 2 Men and 1 in 3 Women," by Zosia Chustecka, Medscape, February 9, 2007.
33. Health: "Non-Hodgkin Lymphoma and Occupational Exposure to Agricultural Pesticide Chemical Groups and Active Ingredients: A Systematic Review and Meta-Analysis Source," by Leah Schinasi and Maria E. Leon, Int J Environ Res Public Health. 2014 Apr.
34. Glyphosate: "Glyphosate induces human breast cancer cells growth via estrogen receptors," by Thongprakaisang S, Thiantanawat A, Rangkadilok N, Surivo T, and Satavivad J, Journal of Food & Chemical Toxicology, June 2013, ncbi.nlm.nih.gov/pubmed/23756170.
35. Birth Defects: "Serious birth defect on the rise, CDC researchers say," by Jen Christensen, CNN, January 22, 2016, https://www.cnn.com/2016/01/22/health/birth-defect-gastroschisis-increase/index.html.
36. Birth Defects: "Roundup and Birth Defects; Is the public being kept in the dark?" by Antoniou, Habib, Howard, Jennings, Leifery, Nodari, Robinson, Fagan, Earth Open Source, June 2011, http://earthopensource.org/earth-open-source-reports/roundup-and-birth-defects-is-the-public-being-kept-in-the-dark/.
37. Glyphosate: "Glyphosate-based herbicides are toxic and endocrine disruptors in human cell lines," by Carla L. Barberis, Cecilia S. Carranza, Stella M. Chiacchiera, and Carina E. Magnoli, Toxicology. 2009 Aug 21;262(3):184-91. doi: 10.1016/j.tox.2009.06.006. Epub 2009 Jun 17.
38. Roundup: "Time and Dose Dependent Effects of Roundup on Human Embryonic and Placenta Cells," by Séralini et al., *Archives of Environmental Contamination and Toxicology*, Arch Environ Contam Toxicol. 2007 Jul;53(1):126-33. Epub 2007 May 4.
39. Roundup: "Roundup disrupts male reproductive functions by triggering calcium-mediated cell death in rat testis and Sertoli cells," by Vera Lúcia de Liz Oliveira Cavallia et al., *Free Radic Biol Med. 2013 Dec;65:335-46. doi: 10.1016/j.freeradbiomed.2013.06.043. Epub 2013 Jun 29.*
40. Infant Mortality: "US has highest first-day infant mortality out of industrialized world, group reports," by Michelle Castillo. CBS News, May 7, 2013, https://www.cbsnews.com/news/us-has-highest-first-day-infant-mortality-out-of-industrialized-world-group-reports/.
41. Fatty Liver Disease: "Multiomics reveal non-alcoholic fatty liver disease in rats following chronic exposure to an ultra-low dose of Roundup herbicide," Robin Mesnage, George Renney, Gilles-Éric Séralini, Malcolm Ward, Michael N. Antoniou, *Scientific Reports,* 09 January 2017.
42. Fetal Exposure: "Pesticide Exposure in Womb Affects I.Q," by Tara Parker-Pope, *New York Times* April 21, 2011, https://well.blogs.nytimes.com/2011/04/21/pesticide-exposure-in-womb-affects-i-q/.
43. National Alliance on Mental Illness, Facts and Numbers: https://namica.org/resources/mental-illness/mental-illness-facts-numbers/.
44. Opioid Epidemic: Vox, "In one year, drug overdoses killed more Americans than the entire Vietnam War did.
45. 2015 was the worst year for drug overdose deaths in US history. Then 2016 came along." by German Lopez, June 8, 2017.
46. https://www.vox.com/policy-and-politics/2017/6/6/15743986/opioid-epidemic-overdose-deaths-2016.

Part Two: UNSTOPPABLE Community

Chapter Four: Trust, Truth, and Community

So Many of Our Kids

1. Dr. Gershon and the gut, "Think Twice: How the Gut's "Second Brain" Influences Mood and Well-Being," by Adam Hadhazy, Scientific American, on February 12, 2010, https://www.scientificamerican.com/article/gut-second-brain/.

The Silent Community

2. Glyphosate: "Glyphosate-based herbicides are toxic and endocrine disruptors in human cell lines," by Céline Gasnier, Coralie Dumont, Nora Benachour, Emilie Clair, Marie-Christine Chagnon, and Gilles-Éric Séralini, Toxicology. 2009 Aug 21;262(3):184-91. doi: 10.1016/j.tox.2009.06.006. Epub 2009 Jun 17.

3. Miscarriage and infant death: "Glyphosate exposure in pregnancy and shortened gestational length: a prospective Indiana birth cohort study," S. Parvez, R. R. Gerona, C. Proctor, M. Friesen, J. L. Ashby, J. L. Reiter, Z. Lui and, P. D. Winchester, Environmental Health, https://doi.org/10.1186/s12940-018-0367-0, 9 March 2018.

Hidden Agendas

4. Donna Farmer edits out miscarriage connection: "Monsanto's Secrets Are Out-Miscarriage Cover-Up Revealed," by Zen Honeycutt, Moms Across America, August 2017, https://www.momsacrossamerica.com/monsanto-secrets-out.

5. Donna Farmer admits glyphosate causes harm when injected: "Admitted: Monsanto's Lead Toxicologist on Glyphosate 'If I Inject It There's a Hazard,'" by Jeffrey Jaxen, May 29, 2017, http://www.jeffereyjaxen.com/blog/admitted-monsantos-lead-toxicologist-on-glyphosate-if-i-inject-it-theres-a-hazard.

6. Alison L. Van Eenennaam and Monsanto: https://www.sourcewatch.org/index.php/Alison_L._Van_Eenennaam.

7. Roundup: "Monsanto Weed Killer Roundup Faces New Doubts on Safety in Unsealed Documents," by Danny Hakim, *New York Times*, March 14, 2017.

8. Cozy ties between Monsanto and EPA: US Right to Know coverage of Baum, Hedlund et al.'s court Case 3:16-md-02741-VC Document 189-1 Filed 03/14/17, https://usrtk.org/wp-content/uploads/2017/03/JessRowlandseries.pdf.

Trusting Farmers, Trusting Nature

9. Glyphosate: "Soil and Environmental Health after Twenty Years of Intensive Use of Glyphosate," by Robert J. Kremer, Advances in Plants & Agriculture, 2017.

10. Farming: "Detection of Glyphosate in Malformed Piglets," by Monika Krüger, Wieland Schrödl, Pedersen, and Awad A. Shehata, December 19, 2012, Environ Anal Toxicol 4:230.

11. Farming: "A long-term toxicology study on pigs fed a combined genetically modified (GM) soy and GM maize diet," by Judy A. Carman, Howard R. Vlieger, Larry J. Ver Steeg, Verlyn E. Sneller, Garth W. Robinson, Catherine A. Clinch-Jones, Julie I. Haynes, John W. Edwards.

12. Monsanto charging 30 percent more for seeds per year: "Cotton Seed Prices Could See Climb from Bayer-Monsanto Merger," by Donna Reynolds, Alabama Cooperative Extension, November 10, 2016.

Scientists Speak the Truth

13. *Poison Spring* author Evaggelos Vallianatos, Ph.D., former EPA analyst.

14. Marion Copley's letter to Jess Rowlands, US Right to Know's coverage of Baum, Hedlund, et al's court Case 3:16-md-02741-VC Document 189-4 Filed 03/14/17, https://usrtk.org/wp-content/

uploads/2017/03/ificankillthis.pdf
15. Glyphosate Review comment-"If I can kill this I should get a medal,"Jess Rowlands: US Right to Know's coverage of Baum, Hedlund, et al's court Case 3:16-md-02741-VC Document 189-4 Filed 03/14/17.

Moms and Science—Bring It On!
16. Mr. Cui Chinese Talk Show Host: https://en.wikipedia.org/wiki/Cui_Yongyuan.
17. Brian A. Federici http://www.entomology.ucr.edu/faculty/federici.html.
18. Soybeans: "Compositional differences in soybeans on the market: glyphosate accumulates in Roundup Ready GM soybeans," by T. Bøhn, M. Cuhra, T. Traavik, M. Sanden, J. Fagan, and R. Primicerio.
19. Bt Toxin used in organic farming: "Bacillus Theringienisis," University of California San Diego, http://www.bt.ucsd.edu/.
20. Double helix in DNA: "Scientists discover double meaning in genetic code," by Stephanie Seiler, University of Washington-Protein and Gene Double Meaning Study, UW Health Sciences & UW Medicine, December 12, 2013. http://www.washington.edu/news/2013/12/12/scientists-discover-double-meaning-in-genetic-code/.
21. Bt Toxin GMOs as Human Gut Pathogen: "The distinct properties of natural and GM cry insecticidal proteins," by Jonathan R. Latham, Madeleine Love and Angelika Hilbeck, Biotechnol Genet Eng Rev. 2017 Apr;33(1):62-96. Epub 2017 Sep 13.
22. Dr. Vandana Shiva eco feminist, Indian scholar, environmental activist, food sovereignty advocate, and anti-globalization author: http://www.navdanya.org/site/.
23. Dr. Michael McNeill farmer educator: http://www.iowacropconsultants.com/vot_mcneilliicca.htm.
24. Gottfried Glockner farmer who confronted Syngenta, Gottfried Glöckner: "How Syngenta destroyed my life for telling the truth about GMOs" by William Engdahl, June 2, 2014.

Chapter Five: A Healthy Community Starts with a Healthy Family
Six Steps to a Healthy Family
1. Antibiotics and gut flora: Dr. Steven Gundry, *The Plant Paradox,* August 23, 2017.
2. Detox: "Oral Application of Charcoal and Humic Acids Influence Selected Gastrointestinal Microbiota, Enzymes, Electrolytes, and Substrates in the Blood of Dairy Cows Challenged with Glyphosate in GMO Feeds," Journal of Environmental & Analytical Toxicology, December 22, 2014. J Environ Anal Toxicol 5:256.
3. Balance Gut Bacteria: Zach Bush, MD http://blog.restore4life.com/university-trained-medical-scientist/.
4. Probiotics: "Mice with Autism Symptoms Decreased with Probiotics," by Kathleen Miles, The Huffington Post Jan 23, 2014.
5. Roundup: "Multiple effects of a commercial Roundup formulation on the soil filamentous fungus Aspergillus nidulans at low doses: evidence of an unexpected impact on energetic metabolism," by Valérie Nicolas, Nathalie Oestreicher, and Christian Vélot.
6. Replenish minerals: from "August Celebration" regarding mineral depletion by Linda Grover: "In 1948 you could buy spinach that had 158 milligrams of iron per hundred grams. But by 1965, the maximum iron they could find had dropped to 27 milligrams. In 1973, it was averaging 2.2 milligrams. That's down from a hundred and fifty. That means today you'd have to eat 75 bowls of spinach to get the same amount of iron that one bowl might have given you back in '48," VitaNet Online April 25, 2004.

Shopping for Healthy Food

7. Organic Food: "Organic versus Non-Organic," A New Evaluation of Nutritional Differences, British Journal of Nutrition, 2012 http://research.ncl.ac.uk/nefg/QOF.

Meat

8. Red Meat: "Processed Red Meats and Cancer One Year Later: Cutting the Risk by Half," by Dr. Joel Kahn, *Huffington Post*, October 24, 2016.
9. Meat: The tenth anniversary edition of *Diet for a Small Planet*, by Frances Moore Lappe states, "According to food geographer Georg Borgstrom, to produce a 1-pound steak requires 2,500 gallons of water" (76).
10. Bioponics: "Board nixes use of carrageenan in organic food production, sends 'bioponics' controversy back to subcommittee," by Cathy Siegner, Food Safety News, November 18, 2016.
11. All about Lectins Precision Nutrition: www.precisionnutrition.com/all-about-lectins.
12. "What Are Nightshade Vegetables?" Dr. Josh Axe, 2018, https://draxe.com/nightshade-vegetables/.

Chapter Six: Toxins in Daily Life

1. Eighty thousand chemicals approved by EPA: Natural Resources Defense Council, https://www.nrdc.org/issues/toxic-chemicals.

Vaccines

2. Vaccine ingredients: https://www.cdc.gov/vaccines/vac-gen/additives.htm.
3. GMOs in the food supply: "GMO Timeline—A History of Genetically Modified Foods," as originally seen on Rosebud Magazine, 2012, with sources added by GMO-Awareness, GMO-Awareness.com, 2011–2014.
4. Seventy-five cents per vaccine is put in fund for vaccines: "Federal program for vaccine-injured children is failing, Stanford scholar says," by Clifton B. Parker, *Stanford News*, July 6, 2015.
5. Vaccine Damages: "Vaccine Court has paid 3.7 billion in damages to families," Health Freedom Idaho, August 16, 2017.
6. Co-Formulants 1,000 times more toxic: "Co-Formulants in Glyphosate-Based Herbicides Disrupt Aromatase Activity in Human Cells Below Toxic Levels," by Nicolas Defarge, Eszter Takács, Verónica Laura Lozano, Robin Mesnage, Joël Spiroux de Vendômois, Gilles-Éric Séralini, and András Székács.
7. Autism: "Is there a link between autism and glyphosate-formulated herbicides?" by James E. Beecham and Stephanie Seneff.
8. Vaccines: Mercola article: "Warn Your Friends and Family: The Fluzone High-Dose Vaccine Is Dangerous," Dr. Joseph Mercola, October 17, 2011.

Protecting Our Animals

9. Dr. Robb: "Veterinarian says pet deaths caused by over-vaccination," by Vicki Batts, Sunday, March 5, 2017.
10. Organic Food: "Organic versus Non-Organic" A New Evaluation of Nutritional Differences. Newcastle University, British Journal of Nutrition, http://research.ncl.ac.uk/nefg/QOF.
11. Goats produced less milk on GMO feed: "Genetically modified soybean in a goat diet: Influence on Kid Performance," by Tudisco, R., et al., Small Ruminant Res. (2015), http://dx.doi.org/10.1016/j.smallrumres.2015.01.023
12. Glyphosate: "EPA Raises Levels of Glyphosate in Food," by Laura Sesana, *Washington Times*, July 5, 2013.
13. Roundup: "Crops Are Drenched with Roundup Pesticide Right Before Harvest." November 17,

2014 by Washington's Blog, http://washingtonsblog.com/2014/11/roundup-dumped-crops-right-harvest.html.
14. Wildlife: "Why Millions of Monarch Butterflies Are Dying in Mexico," by Alicia Graef, EcoWatch, September 7, 2016, https://www.ecowatch.com/monarch-butterflies-mexico-1992151640.html.
15. Pollinator die off: "Save the Bees, Be the solution to help protect bees in crisis," Greenpeace, https://www.greenpeace.org/usa/sustainable-agriculture/save-the-bees/.
16. Insects: "German Nature Reserves Have Lost More Than 75% of Flying Insects," by Lorraine Chow ECOWatch, October 19, 2017, https://www.ecowatch.com/flying-insects-germany-2498472920.html.
17. Decline of birds: Independent, Environment, "'Shocking' decline in birds across Europe due to pesticide use, say scientists 'New figures reveal decline in farmland birds at a level approaching an ecological catastrophe,'" Josh Gabbatiss Science Correspondent Wednesday 21 March 2018, https://www.independent.co.uk/environment/europe-bird-population-countryside-reduced-pesticides-france-wildlife-cnrs-a8267246.html.
18. Extinction: "Timeline of Mass Extinction Events on Earth," by Amber Pariona, World Atlas, April 25, 2017.
19. Extinction: "The Sixth Mass Extinction and Chemicals in the Environment," by Rosemary Mason, JPBC, Volume 15, June 2015 http://www.academia.edu/17783363/The_sixth_mass_extinction_and_chemicals_in_the_environment.
20. Fish: "California's fish population has declined 70% since 1970," CBS8.com October 29, 2015, http://www.cbs8.com/story/30387804/californias-fish-population-has-declined-70-since-1970.
21. Wildlife: "Half of Canada's monitored wildlife is in decline, major study finds," by Ashifa Kassam, *The Guardian*, September 2017.
22. Fish: "Faster Food: Genetically Altered Salmon May Speed to Market," by Jeremy Hsu, LiveScience, September 22, 2010.
23. Wildlife: "Pollution from Hawaii Is Giving Sea Turtles Gross, Deadly Tumors," by Rachel Nuwer, SMARTNEWS, Smithsonian.com, October 2, 2014.
24. Eighty-five percent of oyster beds gone: "World's Oyster Populations Have Declined Precipitously, Study Says," Yale Environment 360, E360 DIGEST, February 3, 2011, https://e360.yale.edu/digest/worlds-oyster-populations-have-declined-precipitously-study-says.
25. Glyphosate: "Glyphosate-based herbicides are toxic and endocrine disruptors in human cell lines," by Céline Gasnier, Coralie Dumont, Nora Benachour, Emilie Clair, Marie-Christine Chagnon, and Gilles-Éric Séralini, Elsevier Toxicology, 2009.
26. Glyphosate disrupts animal reproductive functions: "Roundup disrupts male reproductive functions by triggering calcium-mediated cell death in rat testis and Sertoli cells," by Vera Lúciade, Liz Oliveira Cavalli, Daiane Cattani, Carla Elise Heinz Rieg, Paula Pierozan, Leila Zanatta, Eduardo Benedetti Parisotto, Danilo Wilhelm Filho, Fátima Regina Mena Barreto Silva, Regina Pessoa-Pureur, and Ariane Zamoner.

Part Three: UNSTOPPABLE Leadership

Chapter Seven: Activism

Empowerment in Action

1. Glyphosate: "Argentina: 30,000 Doctors and Health Professionals Demand Ban on Glyphosate," April 19, 2015, by Henry Rowlands, Sustainable Pulse.

Our Role as Americans

2. Tami Monroe-Canal-Feature Interview: March Against Monsanto Founder on the Future, "Pro-Organic vs. Anti-Monsanto" Debate and More by Nick Meyer, July 2, 2013.
3. Fluoride as neurotoxin: "Impact of fluoride on neurological development in children," by T. H. Chan, Harvard, School of Public Health, July 25, 2012.
4. School Lunches: "School Lunches Go Organic. Science supports growing movement," by Aviva Glaser and Michele Roberts, Beyond Pesticides, Vol 6, No 1, 2006.
5. How Do You Have Your Town Go Toxin-Free?: www.momsacrossamerica.org/action.

People in Politics
6. National Toxicology Program: https://ntp.niehs.nih.gov/results/areas/glyphosate/index.html.

Mothers Across the World
7. One in thirty-three children in Philippines with autism: "Shockingly Higher Rates of Autism and Developmental Delays in Asia," by Zen Honeycutt, OCA, March 22, 2017, https://www.organic-consumers.org/news/shockingly-higher-rates-autism-and-developmental-delays-asia#close.
8. Increase of Autism: "1 in 36: ASD Rate Set a New Record High in 2016," Age of Autism on December 01, 2017 at 02:22 PM in Current Affairs, Mark Blaxill, http://www.ageofautism.com/2017/12/autism-1-in-36-asd-rate-set-a-new-record-high-in-2016.html.

Chapter Nine: Speaking to Friends, Family, and Strangers
How to Talk about GMOs and Toxins
1. Uterine Deformities: "Effects of a Glyphosate-Based Herbicide on the Uterus of Adult Ovariectomized Rats," by Jorgelina Varayoud, Milena Durando, Jorge G. Ramos, Maria M. Milesi, Paola I. Ingaramo, Monica Mu-noz-de-Toro, Enrique H.Luque, First published: 27 July 2016, https://doi.org/10.1002/tox.22316.
2. Birth Defects: "Glyphosate Based Herbicides Produce Teratogenic Effects on Vertebrates by Impairing Retinoic Acid Signaling," by Alejandra Paganelli, Victoria Gnazzo, Helena Acosts, Silvia L. Lopez, and Andres E. Carrasco, Laboratorio de Embriologia Molecular, Paraguay, May 20, 2010.
3. Goat Feed: "Genetically modified soybean in a goat diet: Influence on kid performance," by R. Tudiscoa, S. Calabròa, M. I. Cutrignelli , G. Moniello, M. Grossi , V. Mastellonea, P. Lombardi, M. E. Peroa, and F. Infascelli.

Chapter Ten: In the Lion's Den
1. Ecology: "Pesticides in Mississippi air and rain: a comparison between 1995 and 2007," by Majewski MS, Coupe RH, Foreman WT, and Capel PD.
2. Roundup: "Endocrine disruption and cytotoxicity of glyphosate and roundup in human JAr cells in vitro," by Fiona Young, Dao Ho, Danielle Glynn, and Vicki Edwards.
3. Glyphosate: "Glyphosate-based herbicides are toxic and endocrine disruptors in human cell lines," by Céline Gasnier, Coralie Dumont, Nora Benachour, Emilie Clair, Marie-Christine Chagnon, and Gilles-Éric Séralini, Elsevier Toxicology, 2009.
4. Glyphosate: "Glyphosate kills human placental cells which can lead to endocrine disruption (fetal death and deformity)." Integrative Pharmacology, Toxicology and Genotoxicology Integr Pharm Toxicol Gentocicol, 2015 doi: 10.15761/IPTG.1000104 Volume 1(1): 12–19.
5. Glyphosate: "Endocrine disruption and cytotoxicity of glyphosate and roundup in human" JAr cells in vitro Fiona Young, Dao Ho, Danielle Glynn and Vicki Edwards Department of Medical Biotechnology, Flinders University, Adelaide, South Australia, 2018.
6. Harm to testes: "Roundup disrupts male reproductive functions by triggering calcium-mediated

cell death in rat testis and Sertoli cells," by Vera Lúcia de Liz Oliveira Cavalli, Daiane Cattani, Carla Elise Heinz Rieg, Paula Pierozan, Leila Zanatta, Eduardo Benedetti Parisotto, Danilo Wilhelm Filho, Fátima Regina Mena Barreto Silva, Regina Pessoa-Pureur, and Ariane Zamoner, Elsevier, Free Radical Biology and Medicine, 2013.
7. Roundup: "Time- and Dose-Dependent Effects of Roundup on Human Embryonic and Placental Cells," by N. Benachour, H. Sipahutar, S. Moslemi, C. Gasnier, C. Travert, G. E.
8. Glyphosate: "Glyphosate-Based Herbicides Produce Teratogenic Effects on Vertebrates by Impairing Retinoic Acid Signaling," by Alejandra Paganelli, Victoria Gnazzo, Helena Acosta, Silvia L. López, and Andrés E. Carrasco.
9. Autism and Altered Intestinal Bacteria Associated with High Intake of GMO-Foods and Exposure to Weed-Killer, Glyphosate: "Elevated Urinary Glyphosate and Clostridia Metabolites with Altered Dopamine Metabolism in Triplets with Autistic Spectrum Disorder or Suspected Seizure Disorder: A Case Study," William Shaw, Ph.D, imjournal.com Integrative Medicine, February 2017.
10. Glyphosate: "Glyphosate persistence in seawater," by Philip Mercurio, Florita Flores, Jochen F. Mueller, Steve Carter, and Andrew P. Negri, Elsevier, 2014.

Dow, DuPont, and Syngenta Shareholders' Meetings

11. Glyphosate: "EPA completes glyphosate review; findings expected no later than July," by Carey Gillam, Reuters, May 5, 2015.

Corporate Agenda

12. Roundup: "Monsanto and Valent U.S.A. LLC Announce Expanded Partnership in Roundup Ready PLUS Crop Management Solutions," Cision, PR Newswire, August 7, 2017.
13. Thirty-eight weeds now resistant to glyphosate herbicides: "Overview of glyphosate-resistant weeds worldwide," by Ian Heap and Stephen O. Duke, Pest Management Science, Wiley Online Library, November 29, 2017.
14. Shareholders: "Financial Regulation Bill Could Threaten Shareholder Proposal Process," by N. Peter Rasmussen, Bloomberg, Corporate Transactions Blog, Apr 16, 2017.
15. Soil: "UK To Lose Soil Fertility in 30 Years, Says Environment Secretary," by Diana Lupica, Plant Based News, October 25, 2017.
16. Soil: "How Chemical Fertilizers Are Destroying Our Soil and Water," by Dr. Joseph Mercola, Organic Consumers Association, July 2, 2013.
17. Monsanto genetically engineers soil microbes: "Good Riddance, Chemicals: Microbes are Farming's Hot New Pesticides," by Sarah Zhang, Wired Magazine, Science March 21, 2016.
18. DDT still sold in third world countries: "Banned Pesticides Heavily Used in Third World," by Lewis Machipisa, Albion Monitor, November 23, 1996.
19. DDT: "The DDT Story," Pesticide Action Network, http://www.panna.org/resources/ddt-story.

ABOUT THE AUTHOR

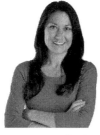

Zen L. Honeycutt is—first and foremost—a mom. She is also an activist, speaker, author, founding executive director of Moms Across America, and cocreator, with Dr. Vandana Shiva, of Mothers Across the World.

Known for being UNSTOPPABLE, Zen makes a practice of going head-to-head with government agencies, big corporations, and anyone who believes that things simply are the way they are and that it's impossible to create change. She knows from experience that anything is possible. Her own story is proof of her beliefs.

Happy to speak to anyone interested in better health for all, she has been featured on ABC, CNN, *The Dr. Oz Show*, the *Wall Street Journal*, C-SPAN, Fox News, Reuter's, *Huffington Post*, and many other media outlets. Zen is available for consulting to nonprofits, organizations, and companies that support the expansion of the organic market and sustainable, toxin-free lifestyles. She has created several successful social media platforms, including the Moms Across America Facebook page, which reaches over a million people a month. Her documentary *Communities Rising* highlights efforts across our nation to transform the food supply.

For years she has been motivating groups around the globe to take action to improve their quality of life, health, and food. Speaking tours have taken her to Australia, New Zealand, Japan, Switzerland, China, Maui, France, The Hague, and all across mainland America.

Zen, formerly of Connecticut and New York City, currently resides in Southern California with Todd, her husband of nineteen years, Ben, Bodee, and Bronson, her three sons, and their dog, Princess Zoe. In her spare time, Zen loves life drawing, swing dancing, spending time at the beach, and singing off-key.

To get in touch with Zen or Moms Across America, visit zenhoneycutt.com, momsacrossamerica.org, or facebook.com/MomsAcrossAmerica.

Made in the USA
San Bernardino, CA
19 May 2018